Scientific Approach to Schizophrenia

Table of Contents

Introduction

Schizophrenia is a chronic psychiatric disorder with a heterogeneous genetic and neurobiological background that influences early brain development, and is expressed as a combination of psychotic symptoms such as hallucinations, delusions and disorganization and motivational and cognitive dysfunctions. The mean lifetime prevalence of the disorder is just below 1%, but large regional differences in prevalence rates are evident owing to disparities in urbanicity and patterns of immigration. Although gross brain pathology is not a characteristic of schizophrenia, the disorder involves subtle pathological changes in specific neural cell populations and in cell communication. Schizophrenia, as a cognitive and behavioural disorder, is ultimately about how the brain processes information. Indeed, neuroimaging studies have shown that information processing is functionally abnormal in patients with first-episode and chronic schizophrenia. Although pharmacological treatments for schizophrenia can relieve psychotic symptoms, such drugs generally do not lead to substantial improvements in social, cognitive and occupational functioning. Psychosocial interventions such as cognitive behavioural therapy, cognitive remediation and supported education and employment have added treatment value, but are inconsistently applied. Given that schizophrenia starts many years before a diagnosis is typically made, the identification of individuals at risk and those in the early phases of the disorder, and the exploration of preventive approaches are crucial.

What is Schizophrenia

Schizophrenia is an incredible example of mental muddle which is exemplified by crumbling of thought processes and emotional receptiveness. It can be straightforwardly acknowledged by auditory hallucinations, paranoid or bizarre illusions, dislocated speech or thinking aptitude pursued by social or occupational dysfunction. The warning signs initiate untimely in the adulthood. The disease is recognized to affect about 1% of the human population with about 2 million patients from the United States unaided. Schizophrenia is also known as split personality disorder and it affects men extra recurrently in contrast to women. A number of aspects play decisive task in aggravating the symptoms of this disorder and these issues are genetic parameters, early environment, neurobiology, physiological and social processes. Some drugs also contribute a petite portion in making the condition of the patient poorer.

In the present scenario researchers are very much spotlighted on the neurobiological factors but no apposite consequence has cropped up. The authentic cause of the disorder is still a contentious concern and the intact argument is centered on the verity that whether the disorder is due to a single cause or other syndromes are also correlated with it. The word schizophrenia has been taken from a Greek word implicating split mind. Antipsychotic medication is usually applied while treating the patients of this disorder as it curbs dopamine and serotonin receptor bustle. Psychotherapy tracked by social and vocational rehabilitation play an imperative role in treatment. In very ruthless cases hospitalization becomes obligatory. The disorder is essentially branded to influence cognition causing setbacks connected with behavior and emotions. Patients also suffer from depression and anxiety disorders. The typical life span of the patient is of 12-15 years after the identification of the disease.

Schizophrenia is a complex syndrome with a heterogeneous combination of symptoms. Characteristic, but by no means exclusive, symptoms of schizophrenia can be divided into 'positive', 'negative' and 'cognitive' categories. Positive symptoms are behaviours and thoughts that are not normally present, such as recurrent psychosis, which is the 'loss of contact with reality' consisting of delusions, hallucinations and disorganized speech and behaviour. The amotivational syndrome is characterized by negative symptoms, which include social withdrawal, affective flattening, anhedonia (the inability to feel pleasure) and diminished initiative and energy. Finally, cognitive symptoms are expressed as a broad set of cognitive dysfunctions. The onset of the illness, although often not recognized as such, is referred to as the prodromal phase (that is, before the manifestation of the first psychotic episode) and consists of a decline in cognitive and social func-tioning, which generally begins in the early adolescent years and precedes the onset of psychotic symptoms by 10years. However, patients are typically not referred for consultation until psychosis presents in late adolescence or early adulthood. The outcome of schizophrenia can range from complete recovery to chronic need of care, and, on average, the life expectancy of those with the disorder is reduced by 20years compared with the general population. Patients with schizophrenia generally experience serious impairments in multiple domains of everyday life, including the ability to maintain social relationships, sustain employment and live independently. These deficits typically persist after patients achieve remission from psychotic symptoms. The abil-ity for patients with schizophrenia to live independently can be achieved for the vast majority of patients using a combination of antipsychotic medication and psychosocial interventions, which increase quality of life (QOL), but have little effect on social and professional functioning. Instead, functional outcomes largely depend on the presence and severity of cognitive and negative symp-toms at disease onset. Thus, several research projects currently focus on psychological, social or pharmacological interventions to reduce cognitive impairments in schizophrenia. The past decade has witnessed an increase in research studies in the field of schizophrenia. First, it has become clear that schizophrenia is much more than a psychotic disorder, and that a renewed focus on cognition is warranted. Second, with the realization that schizophrenia debuts in early adolescences, and not in early adulthood as initially thought, the early identification of individuals at increased risk is now viewed as both clinically and scientifically imperative. Last, progress is rapidly being

Certain groups are at particular risk of the disorder, with various modifiable and non-modifiable risk factors influencing the development of schizophrenia.

History of Schizophrenia : Origination and Meaning

Schizophrenia is a type of mental disorder in which a person suffers from distorted perception of real life and very often losing touch with reality. Originating from the Geek word: schizo (split) and phrene (mind), it is a mental disorder with a long history.

The History of Schizophrenia dated back to around 2000 B.C., when little was known about mental disorders. It was believed that the person who is suffering from mental disturbances has been invaded by an evil spirit and the only way to cure the disorder is by driving out the evil spirit. In those times, there were many types of exorcism method. One was to made patients listen to music in order to drive the evil spirit out, another brutal one see patients skull being drill to provide a way for the spirits to get out.

Schizophrenia as understood by the Egyptians

A mention of mental disorders and their symptoms is there in The Book of Heart, an Egyptian book. The Egyptians believed that the heart and brain are interlinked. Therefore, according to their belief, a person who is suffering from certain mental disorder must be suffering from certain heart problems as well. All the people suffering from Schizophrenia were considered mad and dangerous, in spite of the display of their normal human characteristics at all other times. The only refuges for them were the mental homes. Such misunderstanding stayed for a very long time before researchers came up with a scientific explanation to dispel the misconception.

Evolution in the understanding of Schizophrenia

Initial efforts to understand and record a typical mental behaviors were made in the seventeenth century. Where they started to record and put into place the different types of mental disorders and defined them by one term: dementia praecox. It was not until the nineteenth century before people begin to gain more awareness about diseases and their causes. It was not until the turn of the century before we saw many new medical science breakthrough findings.

Regardless of the progression in medical science, there were few people who were unable to accept the logic and explanation of science and for their benefit continued to commit cruelty towards human race, one such example is the case of World War II. During the World War II Schizophrenia was identified to be a genetic disorder and in order to prevent transmission of the condition from one generation to another and practice selective procreation, mentally disturbed people were killed.

Despite of such pathetic examples in the history of Schizophrenia, psychiatrists, doctors and scientists have never given up hope and have worked day and night for advancement in the understanding of Schizophrenia. Many misconceptions about Schizophrenia have become clear. Today, instead of brutally treating the patients, considering the patients mad and sending them to asylum, society is becoming able to accept the fact that such patients need understanding and sympathy. To help treat and relieve their mental disorder, you need to spend time, show care and affection with proper medication.

Basic Facts

Schizophrenia is a common psychiatric disorder that can affect a person's thinking, emotions, and behaviors. Individuals with this illness will have periods when they have difficulty understanding the reality around them. They may hear voices other people don't hear. They may have unusual thoughts and suspicions, such as believing that other people are reading their minds, controlling their thoughts, or plotting to harm them. These experiences can terrify people with the illness and make them withdrawn or extremely agitated. In addition to symptoms such as hallucinations and delusions, which are also called positive symptoms, nearly all people with schizophrenia have some impairments in their memory, attention, and decision making. These are called cognitive impairments. Some individuals with this illness also have what are called negative symptoms. These can include a lack of expressiveness, low motivation, apathy, an inability to experience pleas- ure, and a disinterest in social relationships. Depression can also be a part of the illness.

Families and Society are affected by Schizophrenia too.

Many people with Schizophrenia have difficulty holding a job or caring for themselves, so they rely on others for help. Some- times symptoms may be so severe that a person needs to be hospitalized.

There are treatments to help improve functioning and relieve many symptoms of schizophrenia. Some individuals re- spond very well to these treatments and can lead rewarding and meaningful lives. Others remain severely disabled by their illness.

Course of Illness

Schizophrenia often first appears during young adulthood (late teens or early twenties for men and late twenties or early thirties for women). The onset of symptoms may be abrupt or gradual, but most people experience some early signs prior to the beginning of active symptoms. These early signs may include depression, social withdrawal, loss of interests, unusual behavior, or decreases in functioning (such as in school, work, or social relationships). These are often the first behaviors to worry family members and friends.

The course of schizophrenia over time varies considerably from person to person. Most individuals experience periods of symptom exacerbation and remission, while others are more chronically ill and maintain a steady level of moderate to severe symptoms and disability over time. Some individuals have a milder course of illness. The positive symptoms of schizophrenia increase during a relapse while negative symptoms and cognitive impairments tend to be more persistent and are present between episodes. Although there is great variability, some generalizations can be made about the long term course of schizophrenia. While many individuals do not return to their prior state of functioning, about one half to two thirds of people with schizophrenia significantly improve or recover, some completely. About one-third of individuals are significantly affected by the disorder and experience frequent hospitalization, and about 10% of these individuals experience long-term institutionalization.

Schizophrenia Clinical Features and Diagnosis

Schizophrenia is a severe and enduring mental health disorder that is often diagnosed in late adolescence or early adulthood. It can present with a wide assortment of symptoms that distort the form and content of thinking and perceptions, which can lead to the development of strange behaviours. Schizophrenia can be chronic or relapsing and remitting. The term "schizophrenia" was used to describe a syndrome of distorted perceptions and behaviours. Today, Schizophrenia is classified into several different subtypes based on presenting symptoms. People with schizophrenia have a lower quality of life than the general population. This may be related to the side effects of medicines, financial difficulties, lack of social support networks and stigma associated with the disorder.

Epidemiology

The World Health Organization estimates that schizophrenia is the 10th most common non-fatal disease worldwide.6 Although the yearly incidence is low (0.015%), due to the chronic nature of the disorder the lifetime prevalence is around 1%. Schizophrenia is more common among men and among immigrants and urban populations. The average age of onset is 18 years for men and 25 years for women. Women also have an increased risk of developing schizophrenia in their mid forties. It has been estimated that in the UK the direct costs of schizophrenia treatment and care amount to £2bn per year. The condition is also associated with indirect costs including: loss of productivity of patients and their carers, criminal justice system costs and benefit payments. People with a diagnosis of schizophrenia are at a higher risk of suicide than those in the general population. Approximately 10% commit suicide the most common cause of premature death in this patient group.

Psychiatric Comorbidity

Psychiatric Comorbidities are freuent among patients with schizophrenia. Substance misuse is also common; conservative estimates suggest at least half of patients are affected. Comorbid depression occurs in 50% of patients. Anxiety disorders (particularly panic disorder, post-traumatic stress disorder and obsessive compulsive disorder) can also be present to varying degrees.

Epidemiology Morbidity and Mortality

The average lifetime prevalence of narrowly defined schizophrenia, for instance, according to the diagnostic criteria from the Diagnostic and Statistical Manual of Mental Disorders, Fourth Edition (DSM-IV), is just under 1%. The most detailed study on schizophrenia prevalence was conducted in Finland and found a rate of 0.87%6. However, prevalence rates vary geographically by up to fivefold. People with schizophrenia have, on average, a shorter life than the rest of the population. A systematic review of mortality studies reported that the standardized mortality ratio was 2.6, with suicide being the main contribu-tor early in the course of the illness and cardiovascular disease the main contributor in later years. The persistently high rate of cigarette smoking among people with schizophrenia, the increased likelihood they will have an unhealthy lifestyle and the obesity-promoting effects of antipsychotic drugs contribute to metabolic syndrome, diabetes and excess cardiovascular and respiratory deaths among these patients. Disappointingly, the disparity in life expectancy between people with schizophrenia and the general population has been worsening Paternal age.

Men who are older when fathering a child have a greater chance of having a child who develops schizophrenia than younger men; however, whether this risk is due to psychological or biological factors is unclear. For example, men with a schizotypal personality might be more likely to marry later, or, alternatively, older men might harbour more risk increasing mutations as a result of repeated mitosis in progenitors of sperm cells. The evidence currently favours the idea that the association between late fatherhood and schizotypal personality is the predominant driver of this effect. Sex. Schizophrenia is generally reported to be slightly more frequent in men than in women, with a risk ratio of 1.4/1. The disorder is also more severe in men. In addition, men tend to develop severe schizophrenia earlier than women; the peak age of onset of frank psychotic symptoms is 20–24years in men, but 5 or more years later in women13–15. Urban environment. Schizophrenia is most common in disadvantaged areas of inner cities, This association was recently replicated in an epidemiological study in England, the Aetiology and Ethnicity in Schizophrenia and Other Psychoses (AESOP) study, which reported that the incidence of schizophrenia in the smaller cities of Nottingham and Bristol was less than half of that in London. The highest rates of people with schizophrenia in London were in areas with the lowest social cohesion, a finding that was also reported in the original Chicago study. Scandinavian studies have shown increased incidence of schizophrenia in people born or raised in urban areas compared with those born or raised in rural areas. For example, a Danish study showed that the risk of developing schizophrenia was greater in those not only born but also raised exclusively in large cities compared with individuals who had experienced less urbanized environments.

Migration status. An increased incidence of schizophrenia has been demonstrated among many migrant groups compared with those comprising individuals who do not have a personal or family history of migration. However, recent literature has focused on black migrants to European countries who show much higher rates of schizophrenia than white or Asian migrants to Europe, or indeed migrants to other continents. For example, the AESOP study showed that in the population of black migrants and their children there was at least a sixfold greater incidence of schizophrenia than in the white British population. In support of this conclusion, in this study diagnosis was made blind to ethnicity to exclude the contribution of possible racial or cultural bias by clinicians. Interestingly, studies of the relatives of African Caribbean patients with schizophrenia who live in England have shown that the risk of developing the dis order is much lower in those siblings living in the Caribbean than in those who reside in England. Such findings suggest the influence of an environmental factor in the European host country but not in the country of origin. Ethnic density also seems to be important; as the relative proportion of non white minorities in a neighbourhood increases, the risk of schizophrenia in the minority population decreases. Thus, lack of social support or increased exposure to discrimination might operate to increase the risk of develop ing the disorder, especially in areas with only a small minority population. Drug abuse. Persistent abuse of amphetamine, methamphetamine and cocaine, as well as cathinone-derived 'legal highs' can produce a state that is almost identical to that of paranoid schizophrenia. Moreover, experimental administration of cannabis or its active ingredient tetrahydrocannabinol can precipitate transient psychotic symptoms and smoking cannabis is known to exacerbate existing psychotic illness. In addition, a series of prospective studies have shown that young people who heavily use cannabis have an increased risk of subsequent schizo-phrenia and that this relationship is dosedependent. The risk is greater in those who start cannabis use in early adolescence than in those who start use later in life and in those using high-potency varieties of cannabis. In recent years, even more potent synthetic cannabinoids (spice) have become widely available over the Internet and have been linked to acute psychotic reactions. Social adversity. A range of childhood adversities including physical abuse, sexual abuse, maltreatment and bullying are associated with increased risk of later schizophrenia. People with psychosis also report an increased rate of particularly intrusive life events, such as assault, before the onset of illness. Whether these environmental factors are independent risk factors is debated. Evidence supporting their independence comes from PET studies showing that most factors have an effect on striatal dopamine synthesis. However, it is possible that people who are genetically predisposed to schizophrenia might be more likely to be exposed to social risk factors, such as being bullied. Resolution of this ☐uestion should be achievable by examining the polygenic risk score, which is produced by summing the risk values of the various genetic loci that have been associated with schizophrenia among people experiencing these adversities.Mechanisms/pathophysiologySchizophrenia is hypothesized to be the result of a complex interplay between genetic and environmental risk factors that influence early brain development and the trajectory of biological adaptation to life experiences. Archival post-mortem studies of patients who had been diagnosed with schizophrenia suggest that the brains of these individuals have gross cellular abnormalities, but these findings have not been confirmed by rigorous controlled investigations over the past two decades, indi-cating that gross brain pathology is not a characteristic of schizophrenia. Recent studies have focused instead on the molecular signatures of a moresubtle pathology that primarily involves the functional state of specific cell populations and the architecture of cell to cell communication. Although some replicated findings that are suggestive of a molecular neuropathology of schizophrenia have been reported, this work is fundamentally hindered by the limitations of determining causality in this context, thus making it difficult to disambiguate what is related to the state of illness and the epiphenomena of illness such as the effects of treatment, disease chronicity and co-morbidity from basic mechanisms that lead to illness. Pharmacological studies of psychotogenic and antipsychotic drugs have fuelled hypotheses focused on neurotransmitter mechanisms, but these also have been difficult to translate into explanations of the complex clinical syndrome.

Schizophrenia Facts and Myths

Schizophrenia is one of the least culturally understood mental disorders. For example, a common belief is that schizophrenia means split personality; which it doesn't.. It actually means "split mind" from the Greek "schizo" meaning split and "phrene" meaning mind. It was created to describe the type of thinking that someone suffering from schizophrenia exhibited, not multiple personalities. The original term for schizophrenia was "dementia praecox" which means "early dementia." This comes from Dr. Emile Kraepelin who was one of the first to recognize the disorder. The name was to distinguish the disorder from late in life mental disorders such as Alzheimer's. The reason for the many technical names for different disorders is that scientists often do not have a full understanding of the causes of mental diseases and can only classify them by symptoms.

The cause of schizophrenia is still unknown, but its affects on the brain are clear in numerous tests, including MRI. So, schizophrenia can be easily diagnosed with the proper e□uipment. While the cause is still a mystery, there are indications that both genetics and brain chemistry play a role. Another important factor is drug abuse. Drugs like nicotine, marijuana, cocaine and alcohol all have an effect and the abuse of such substances can greatly impede treatment. So, it's important to ensure that schizophrenic patients are kept strictly away from recreational drugs.

Although those with a family history of schizophrenia are more likely to develop it, depression, chronic stress, anxiety and traumatic life events can also trigger the onset of the disorder.

Visual and auditory hallucinations are a feature of schizophrenia, although not in every case. Other significant symptoms are the inability to rationally assess the environment or to rationally understand interactions with other people, which may result in extreme paranoia and lack of trust.

Other symptoms include apathy, poor concentration, withdrawal, difficulty in speaking or movement disorders or a poor ability to express emotions. Nevertheless, it should be kept in mind that other disorders, even very mild ones, can cause some of these symptoms. And so, the symptoms alone do not necessarily signify schizophrenia. People should avoid self-diagnosis. And it should be remembered that one of the hallmarks of schizophrenia is the inability to notice the disorder in oneself. So, if you think that you have schizophrenia, you probably don't. When in doubt, consult a professional.

There are five subtypes of schizophrenia. These are the Paranoid subtype which is typified by delusions of persecution and conspiracy along with auditory hallucinations. Those who suffer from this subtype can often appear normal, or at least what is accepted as normal.

There is Disorganized Schizophrenia which exhibits disorganized thinking and difficulty in performing normal tasks such as bathing and dressing. While symptoms of delusion and hallucination may exist in this subtype, they are not as severe. The other three types are Catatonic, Residual and Undifferentiated.

Diagnosis of schizophrenia usually involves a psychological evaluation including collecting information on the individuals mental health, information on his or her family, understanding the patients medical situation, such as what prescription drugs they might be taking, as well as social and cultural influences. Lab tests are also performed including a complete blood count (CBC), imaging of the brain through MRI and CTs and screening for drugs and alcohol.

Anti-psychotics are presently the best form of treatment, as they help balance neurotransmissions within the brain. But they do have side effects, including weight gain and tremors.

The person diagnosed with schizophrenia will also need the attendance, guidance and understanding of family members if he or she is to get better.

Types of Schizophrenia

There are five types of schizophrenia, They are categorized by the types of symptoms the person exhibits when they are assessed:

> Paranoid Schizophrenia

> Disorganized Schizophrenia

> Catatonic Schizophrenia

> Undifferentiated Schizophrenia

> Residual Schizophrenia

A woman suffering from paranoid schizophrenia is distressed.

Paranoid Schizophrenia

Paranoid type schizophrenia is distinguished by paranoid behavior, including delusions and auditory hallucinations. Paranoid behavior is exhibited by feelings of persecution, of being watched, or sometimes this behavior is associated with a famous or noteworthy person a celebrity or politician, or an entity such as a corporation. People with paranoid type schizophrenia may display anger, anxiety, and hostility. The person usually has relatively normal intellectual functioning and expression of affect.

A young woman pours a pot of spaghetti on her head.

Disorganized Schizophrenia

A person with disorganized type schizophrenia will exhibit behaviors that are disorganized or speech that may be bizarre or difficult to understand. They may display inappropriate emotions or reactions that do not relate to the situation at hand. Daily activities such as hygiene, eating, and working may be disrupted or neglected by their disorganized thought patterns.

A man is in a catatonic state.

Catatonic Schizophrenia

Disturbances of movement mark catatonic type schizophrenia. People with this type of schizophrenia may vary between extremes: they may remain immobile or may move all over the place. They may say nothing for hours, or they may repeat everything you say or do. These behaviors put these people with catatonic type schizophrenia at high risk because they are often unable to take care of themselves or complete daily activities.

A young man with undifferentiated schizophrenia wears a tinfoil hat while staring into a TV.

Undifferentiated Schizophrenia

Undifferentiated type schizophrenia is a classification used when a person exhibits behaviors which fit into two or more of the other types of schizophrenia, including symptoms such as delusions, hallucinations, disorganized speech or behavior, catatonic behavior.

A schizophrenic girl's reflection shows her inner turmoil.

Residual Schizophrenia

When a person has a past history of at least one episode of schizophrenia, but the currently has no symptoms (delusions, hallucinations, disorganized speech or behavior) they are considered to have residual type schizophrenia. The person may be in complete remission, or may at some point resume symptoms.

What Causes Schizophrenia?

Both genetic as well as environmental factors play a strategic role in the development of schizophrenia. People with family history of the disease are at the risk of getting distressed with the disease in near future. However, the guesstimates of heritability vary due to difficulty in separating the genetic as well as environmental factors while identifying the disease. According to an estimate about 40% of the mono-zygotic twins are at the risk of getting infected with this disease. Many genes are associated with development of every symptom of the disorder. A number of genome wide associations like zinc finger protein 804A, NOTCH4 and protein loci are found to be linked. There appears a momentous overlap between the genetics of schizophrenia and bipolar disorder. The environmental factors that are linked with schizophrenia include living environment, prenatal stressors and drug intake. Social isolation and immigration related to social adversity, racial discrimination, family dysfunction, unemployment, and poor housing conditions also play a crucial role in the development of this disorder. Childhood factors like sexual abuse and any trauma can result in schizophrenia in the adulthood.

A number of drugs namely cocaine, cannabis and amphetamines also contribute in the development of schizophrenia. Individuals suffering from schizophrenia normally consume drugs in order to cope up with depression, loneliness, boredom and anxiety. Cannabis is generally associated with increasing the risk of development of a psychotic disorder. Frequent use of this drug generally doubles the risk of getting affected with schizophrenia and psychosis. Excessive intake of cocaine and amphetamine can also increase the risk of schizophrenia. Other factors like hypoxia and infection, stress or malnutrition in the mother during fetal development can somewhat increase the risk of schizophrenia in the baby in later stages of life. Studies have indicated that the people suffering from schizophrenia are generally born in the months of winter and spring and are at the risk of getting infected with viral diseases more frequently. The percentage of such individuals varies from 5-8%

Causes

There is no simple answer to what causes schizophrenia because several factors play a part in the onset of the disorder. These include: a genetic or family history of schizophrenia, environmental stressors and stressful life events, and biological factors.

Research shows that the risk for schizophrenia results from e influence of genes acting together with environmental factors. A family history of schizophrenia does not necessarily ean children or other relatives will develop the disorder. However, studies have shown that schizophrenia does run in families. Others believe the environment plays a key role in whether someone will develop schizophrenia. Some of the environmental factors believed to be linked to schizophrenia are malnutrition before birth, obstetric complications, poverty, and substance use. Cannabis use, especially before age 15, has been identified as a big risk factor. Stressful life events, such as family conflict, early parental loss or separation, and physical or sexual abuse, are also associated with the illness.

An imbalance of the neurotransmitters dopamine and glu- tamate is also linked to schizophrenia. Neurotransmitters are brain chemicals that communicate information throughout the brain and body. However, the exact role of these neurotrans mitters in schizophrenia is unclear. No single cause of schizophrenia has been identified, but several factors have been shown to be associated with its onset. Men and women have an e ual chance of developing this mental illness across the lifespan, although the onset for men is often earlier.

Genetic factors

A predisposition to schizophrenia can run in families. In the general population, only one percent of people develop it over their lifetime, but if one parent has schizophrenia, the children have a 10 percent chance of developing the condition and a 90 percent chance of not developing it.

Biochemical factors

Certain biochemical substances in the brain are believed to be involved in schizophrenia, especially a neurotransmitter called dopamine. One likely cause of this chemical imbalance is the person's genetic predisposition to the illness. Complications during pregnancy or birth that cause structural damage to the brain may also be involved.

Family Relationships

No evidence has been found to support the suggestion that family relationships cause the illness. However, some people with schizophrenia are sensitive to any family tension, which for them may be associated with recurrent episodes.

Stress

It is well recognised that stressful incidents often precede the onset of schizophrenia. These may act as precipitating events in vulnerable people. People with schizophrenia often become anxious, irritable and unable to concentrate before any acute symptoms are evident. This can cause problems with work or study and relationships to deteriorate. Often these factors are then blamed for the onset of the illness when, in fact, the illness itself has caused the stressful event. It is not, therefore, always clear whether stress is a cause or a result of schizophrenia.

Alcohol and other drug use Harmful alcohol and other drug use, particularly cannabis and amphetamine use, may trigger psychosis in people who are vulnerable to developing schizophrenia. While substance use does not cause schizophrenia, it is strongly related to relapse.

People with schizophrenia are more likely than the general population to use alcohol and other drugs, and this is detrimental to treatment.

A considerable proportion of people with schizophrenia have been shown to smoke, which contributes to poor physical health.

- ➢ Biological for example family history (a genetic cause is suggested, but no single gene has been found to be responsible and it is more likely that there are small changes in several genes) or brain injury (caused by birth trauma or fetal exposure to infection)
- ➢ Social such as low socioeconomic status, poor housing, social isolation, loss of cultural identity and discrimination
- ➢ Psychological including early living environment and stressful life events

Symptoms of Schizophrenia

An individual diagnosed with schizophrenia may complain of hallucinations, delusions, disorganized thinking and speech. Disorganized speech includes loss of ability to speak clear sentences. Social withdrawal, sloppiness of dressing and hygiene, loss of motivation and judgment power are common in schizophrenia. Loss of responsiveness and impairment in social cognition are very common in this disorder. Social isolation is the symptom of paranoia. The person may become mute, may show purposeless agitation showing signs of catatonia. Late adolescence and early adulthood are the peak periods at which an individual is at higher risk of getting affected with schizophrenia. Data have shown that in 40% of men and 23% of women the symptoms of schizophrenia generally arise at the age of 19.

Schizophrenia symptoms are classified into two groups: Positive and Negative.

Positive symptoms are those which cause an excess or distortion of normal function, including:

> Delusions: delusions can be somatic (involving false beliefs about physical illnesses), grandiose (containing beliefs of self importance and having special powers or abilities) or paranoid (where there are beliefs of persecution) Social isolation might contribute to the development of schizophrenia

> Hallucinations: hallucinations can be auditory, tactile, visual, olfactory or gustatory, characterised by experiences when there are no external stimuli

> Disorganised speech and behaviour

> Thought disorders thought disorder is characterised by disorganised speech, which is believed to be due to abnormal thoughts; thoughts can be blocked (where little or no thoughts occur), or can appear to have been inserted into, or withdrawn from, the mind by others

> Ideas of reference ideas of reference occur when a person believes that certain external phenomena such as TV, radio or newspaper articles are reporting about them or talking directly to them (ideas of reference can also be considered

delusions if there are beliefs that external happenings relate directly to the individual)

Negative symptoms are those that lead to a decrease or loss of normal function, including lack of emotion, apathy, poor or non existent social functioning, lack of motivation, reduced speech, lack of initiative, slow movements and poor self-care.

It is common for people with schizophrenia to lack insight to such an extent that they do not believe they are ill.

Symptoms vary from person to person, and commonly include:

➢ hearing or seeing things that are not real (hallucinations)

➢ having very strange beliefs (delusions)

➢ unusual thinking and speech

➢ having problems thinking clearly

➢ not being able to make decisions and having trouble making plans

➢ having trouble interpreting other people's emotions and motives

➢ suicidal thoughts.

Some symptoms are described as 'positive' and others as 'negative'. Common 'positive' symptoms are hallucinations and delusions. (These are called 'positive' because they are extra experiences that are not part of normal experience). Common 'negative' symptoms are: a loss of enjoyment of things, being unable to feel emotions, loss of interest in being with other people, and not being bothered to do anything. (These are called 'negative' because something is missing).

Pattern of Symptoms

Times when symptoms worsen are called relapses. When symptoms improve or disappear, it's called remission. When delusions and hallucinations occur or get worse, the person may have trouble with everyday tasks, thinking clearly, solving problems or making decisions. They may be unable to control their emotions or to get on normally with family, friends or other people, including their health care team.

What are the first signs?

Before the signs of psychosis become obvious and schizophrenia can be diagnosed, most people have early stage symptoms. Symptoms can include:

- ➤ changes in normal behaviour, such as work or schoolwork getting worse
- ➤ no longer wanting to spend time with friends
- ➤ dropping out of normal activities
- ➤ beginning to have unusual beliefs hearing sounds that other people can't hear.

Schizophrenia cannot be diagnosed this early, but it means the person is at high risk of developing schizophrenia.

The early stage is like a warning not everyone who has these symptoms will go on to develop a psychosis such as schizophrenia. Some people with the same symptoms may go on to develop another mental illness such as bipolar disorder or anxiety, or be at increased risk of self harm.

It is important to recognise something is not right and get help. Early treatment can delay symptoms of psychosis.

Mechanisms Associated with Schizophrenia

A number of studies have been carried out to find out the link between altered brain function and schizophrenia. The most commonly agreed hypothesis is the dopamine hypothesis which emphasizes that schizophrenia is the result of misfiring of the dopaminergic neurons. A number of psychological interpretations are also thought be responsible for the development of this disorder. Cognitive biases have been identified exclusively in the conditions of confusion and stress. Some cognitive features may lead to memory loss. Recent studies have indicated that the patients of schizophrenia are emotionally responsive to stressful conditions as well as to negative stimuli and such symptoms may worsen the state of the victim. Delusional beliefs and psychotic experiences may also make the condition of the patient poor.

The diagnosis of schizophrenia indicates changes in both brain structure and brain chemistry. Studies using the neurophysiological tests and brain imaging techniues like fMRI and PET have shown functional changes in the brain activity especially of the frontal lobes, temporal lobes and hippocampus. Changes in the brain volume particularly of the frontal cortex and the temporal lobes have been noticed. Since the neural circuits are altered, schizophrenia is sometimes considered as a collection of neuro developmental disorders. While dealing with the mechanism of this disorder much consideration is given to the function of dopamine in the meso limbic pathway of brain. This focus has largely resulted from the accidental finding that the phenothiazine drugs bear the potential of blocking the dopamine function so can help to diminish the psychotic symptoms. It is also supported by the fact that amphetamines which trigger dopamine release can intensify psychotic symptoms. The dopamine hypothesis points out that excessive release of the D2 receptors are the actual cause of schizophrenia.

In the present scenario much focus is centered on the neurotransmitter glutamate and reduced function of NMDA glutamate receptor in schizophrenia. The postmortem of brains of patients of schizophrenia has shown abnormally low levels of glutamate receptors and glutamate blocking drugs can enhance cognitive problems. Reduction in the activity of glutamate can also affect the activity of frontal lobes and the hippocampus. Dopamine function is also known to be affected due to reduction in glutamate activity. Positive symptoms however, fail to respond to the glutamatergic medication.

The symptoms of schizophrenia fall into three broad cate- gories: positive symptoms, negative symptoms, and cognitive symptoms.

POSITIVE SYMPTOMS:

Positive symptoms refer to thoughts, perceptions, and behaviors that are present in people with schizophrenia, but ordinarily absent in other people. These symptoms can come and go. Sometimes they are severe, and and sometimes they are hardly noticeable.

➢ Auditory: Hearing things that other people cannot hear. Many people with the disorder hear voices. The voices may talk to the person about his or her behavior, order the person to do things, or warn the person of danger. Sometimes the voices talk to each other.

➢ Visual: Seeing things that are not there or that other people cannot see.

➢ Tactile: Feeling things that other people don't feel or feeling something is touching their skin that isn't there.

➢ Olfactory: Smelling things that other people cannot smell, or not smelling the same thing that other people do smell.

➢ Gustatory: Tasting things that are not there.

> Delusions: Delusions are false beliefs that are held in spite of invalidating evidence. People hold these beliefs strongly and usually cannot be "talked out" of them. The content of the delusions may include a variety of themes. Some examples include:

> Delusions of persecution: The belief that they (or someone close to them) are being plotted or discriminated against, spied on, threatened, attacked or deliberately victimized.

> Delusions of reference: When an individual attaches special personal meaning to actions of others or to various objects and events when there is no information to confirm this. The person may believe that certain gestures, comments, or other environmental cues are specifically directed at him or her. For ex- ample, it may seem as if special personal messages are being communicated to them through the TV, radio, or other media.

> Somatic delusions: False beliefs about their body. For example, that a terrible physical illness exists or that something foreign is inside or passing through their body.

> Delusions of grandeur: The belief that they are very special or have special powers or abilities.

> Delusions of control: The belief that their feelings, thoughts, and actions are being controlled by other people.

> Thought disorders: Thought disorders are unusual or dysfunctional ways of thinking. One form of thought disorder is called "disorganized thinking." This is when a person has trouble organizing his or her thoughts or connecting them logically. They may string words together in an incoherent way that is hard to understand, often referred to as a "word salad." The person may make "loose

associations," where they rapidly shift from one topic to an unrelated topic, making it very difficult to follow their conversation. "Thought blocking" may occur in which the person stops speaking abruptly in the middle of a thought. When asked why he or she stopped talking, the person may say that it felt as if the thought had been taken out of his or her head. A person with a thought disorder might make up meaningless words, or "neologisms," or perseverate which means to persistently repeat words or ideas.

NEGATIVE SYMPTOMS:

Negative symptoms are the ab- sence of thoughts, perceptions, or behaviors that are ordinarily present in other people. These symptoms are often stable throughout much of the person's life.

- ➤ Affective flattening: Affective flattening is characterized by a reduction in the range of emotional expressiveness, including limited or unresponsive facial expression, poor eye contact, and reduced body language. The expressiveness of the person's face, voice tone, and gestures may be reduced or restricted. However, this does not mean that the person is not reacting to his or her environment or having feelings.
- ➤ Alogia: Alogia, or poverty of speech, is the lessening of speech fluency and productivity. The person may have difficulty or be unable to speak and may give short, empty replies to questions.
- ➤ Avolition: Avolition is the difficulty or inability to begin and persist in goal directed behavior. It is often mistaken for apparent disinterest. The person may not feel motivated to pursue goals and activities. They may have little sense of

purpose in their lives and have few interests. They may feel lethargic or sleepy, and have trouble following through on even simple plans.

➤ Anhedonia: Anhedonia is defined as the inability to experience pleasure from activities one used to find enjoyable. For example, the person may not enjoy watching a sunset, going to the movies, or having close relationships with other people.

COGNITIVE SYMPTOMS:

Cognition refers to mental processes that allow us to perform day to day functions, such as the ability to pay attention, to remember, and to solve problems. Cognitive impairments are considered a core feature of schizophrenia and contribute to difficulties in work, social relationships, and inde- pendent living. Some examples of cognitive symptoms in schizophrenia include: trouble concentrating or paying attention, poor memory, slow thinking, and poor ex- ecutive functioning. Executive functions include the ability to plan, solve problems, and grasp abstract concepts.

Similar Psychiatric Disorders

Schizophrenia shares symptoms with some other psychiatric disorders. Prominent psychotic symptoms seen in schizophrenia are similar to those seen in other psychotic disorders, such as Schizoaffective Disorder, Schizophreni- form Disorder, and Brief Psychotic Disorder. Symptoms of schizophrenia may also overlap with symptoms of Bipolar Disorder. Individuals with schizophrenia may experience mood disturbances seen in Bipolar Disorder, including mania and depression. Schizophrenia must be distinguished from a Psychotic Disorder due to a General Medical Condition, where psychotic symptoms are judged to be the direct conse☐uence of a general medical condition. Schizophrenia must also be distinguished from a Substance Induced Psychotic Disorder, in which psychotic symptoms are judged to be the direct conseＤuence of drug abuse, medication, or toxin exposure.

How Is Schizophrenia Diagnosed?

The diagnosis of schizophrenia is made both by ruling out other medical disorders that can cause the behavioral symptoms (exclusion), and by observation of the presence of characteristic symptoms of the disorder. The doctor will look for the presence of delusions, hallucinations, disorganized speech or behavior, and/or negative symptoms, along with social withdrawal and/or dysfunction at work or in daily activities for at least six months. The doctor may use physical examination, psychological evaluation, laboratory testing of blood, and imaging scans to produce a complete picture of the patient's condition. A mental health professional diagnoses a patient.

Mental health screening and evaluation is an important part of the diagnosis process for schizophrenia. Many other mental illnesses such as bipolar disorder, schizoaffective disorder, anxiety disorders, severe depression, and substance abuse may mimic symptoms of schizophrenia. A doctor will perform an assessment to rule out these other conditions.

Schizophrenia Treatment - Medications

Antipsychotic medications are the first line treatment for many patients with schizophrenia. Medications are often used in combination with other types of drugs to decrease or control the symptoms associated with schizophrenia. Some antipsychotic medications include:

- olanzapine (Zyprexa)

- risperidone (Risperdal)

- quetiapine (Seroquel)

- ziprasidone (Geodon)

- aripiprazole (Abilify)

- paliperidone (Invega)

Diagnosis

Schizophrenia is diagnosed using the International Classification of Diseases Version 10 (ICD-10) criteria.

For a diagnosis to be made there must be clear evidence of either:

- One of the following hallucinations, delusions or thought disorder
- Two of the following catatonia, negative symptoms or a consistent change in personal behaviour

These symptoms must be present for the majority of a one month period.Generally, a diagnosis of schizophrenia will not be made based on a single episode of psychosis. This is because psychosis can occur as part of a number of different mental health conditions or be due to another cause.The onset of the first episode of psychosis of schizophrenia is usually preceded by a prodromal phase. This phase includes symptoms that can cause a deterioration in functioning, such as reduced concentration and attention, reduced drive and motivation, sleep disturbance and anxiety.

Young people often fail to complete further education and become isolative and socially withdrawn. Delay in diagnosing and treating first episode psychosis increases the risk of more severe longterm positive and negative symptoms.

The ICD criteria are also used to classify a patient with schizophrenia based on his or her prominent symptoms at presentation. For example, paranoid schizophrenia has prominent symptoms of paranoid delusions accompanied by auditory hallucinations.

Differential Diagnoses

Some medical conditions can present as psychosis. Thought disorder, delusions, visual and auditory hallucinations and paranoia have been documented with long standing untreated hypothyroidism and hyperthyroidism. Olfactory hallucinations are commonly experienced in temporal lobe epilepsy. Systemic lupus erythematosus, central nervous system tumours, migraines, diabetes, human immunodeficiency virus, head injury and delirium have also all been associated with psychotic symptoms.

There are a number of medicines that can induce psychosis. Levodopa (the amino acid precursor of dopamine) and dopamine agonists such as bromocriptine and pergolide can all cause psychotic symptoms. Furthermore, psychotic symptoms can be caused or worsened by some medicines, including antimuscarinics, some antiinfectives (eg, isoniazid), betablockers, corticosteroids and amphetamines. Psychoactive substances (such as alcohol, hallucinogens, opioids and cannabis) have also been associated with psychotic symptoms.

Cannabis One of the pharmacological effects of cannabis is to increase dopamine release in the brain. As already discussed, an overactivity of dopamine is considered to be the neurochemical basis for schizophrenia. Drug induced psychosis is a commonly observed syndrome and there are concerns about the long term effects of cannabis use on the risk of developing schizophrenia. Recent research has indicated that heavy cannabis users have a sixfold increased risk of developing schizophrenia compared with non users.

Baseline tests A range of baseline tests should be carried out for those with a suspected diagnosis of schizophrenia to exclude any physical conditions that could account for the psychotic symptoms. These should include:

> Thyroid function tests to assess for hyper or hypothyroidism

> Liver function tests to assess alcohol use

> Blood sugar level to assess for diabetes

> Urine drug screening to rule out (or identify) substance misuse

Diagnosis and screeningDiagnosis of schizophrenia is made on the basis of operational criteria, such as those documented in DSM or International Statistical Classification of Diseases and Related Health Problems (ICD). These criteria take into account characteristic positive, negative and cognitive symptoms of schizophrenia along with symptom duration, their effect on social and occupational function-ing and the potential contribution of other psychiatric conditions, mood disorders and substance abuse issues. The high heritability of schizophrenia suggests that, in principle, genetic data might inform risk prediction, diagnostics and possibly stratification approaches to treatment selection. However, given that heritability is not 100%, for the general population of patients, genetics is unlikely to provide definitive risk prediction or diagnostic discrimination. Approximately chromosomal loci containing schizophrenia susceptibility alleles have been identified, most of which (n = 108) were found by genome wide association studies. These loci contain risk alleles with freⓊuencies of ≥1%, and each individual allele confers only a small amount of risk, with allelic odds ratios of approximately ≤1.1. Despite the n umber of implicated loci, cumulatively, Criteria for schizophrenia: The criteria for Schizophrenia from the Diagnostic and Statistical Manual of Mental Disorders, two or more of the following symptoms for >1 month unless treated successfully include delusions; hallucinations; disorganized speech; disorganized or catatonic behaviour; and negative symptoms, such as affective flattening or loss of initiative B criterion: level of functioning is significantly decreased in work, personal relationships and/or personal care C criterion: symptoms of the disorder last ≥6months D criterion: exclusion of schizoaffective disorder, unipolar and bipolar affective disorder E criterion: symptoms cannot be attributed to the use of drugs or medication, or to a somatic disorder F criterion: in the case of a preexisting autism spectrum disorder, at least 1 month with prominent hallucinations or delusions

3.5% of the variance in liability to schizophrenia. One way of capturing more of the variance is through polygenic risk profile scoring (RPS). In RPS, alleles that meet some Pvalue threshold for an association are classified as risk alleles. Risk profile scores are then assigned to individuals based on the number of risk alleles carried that have been weighted by their esti-mated effect size. RPS currently captures about 7% of the liability for schizophrenia in populations of European ancestry, a level that is far short of a clinically useful test. Moreover, the predictive power in non European ancestry populations, particularly of African origin, is even lower. In principle, 25–33% of liabi lity might ultimately be indexed by RPS, but modelling suggests that, as sample sizes increase, accessing this variance will become progressively incremental. Fuller coverage of common variation on genome arrays might boost the information captured by RPS by perhaps another 5 percentage points. Other possible gains might come from allowing for interactive effects. These effects clearly exist at the molecular level, but whether this has the potential to significantly enhance the measured vari ance in liability has been disputed for decades. For now, we can only note that there is no strong evidence for nonadditive effects in genomewide analyses of psychosis or between pairs of genome wide significant schizophrenia loci, although the analyses so far certainly do not preclude these or higher order interactions. RPS and other analogous approaches have revealed a substantial overlap between schizophrenia and both major depressive disorder and bipolar disorder and, to a lesser extent, with attention deficit/hyperactivity disorder (ADHD). Findings such as these, as well as non specificity with respect to other indices or risks, have led to calls for novel ways of classifying psychiatric disorders on the basis of, for example, symptom profiles, cognitive measures or brain imaging variables. The hope is that these might index pathogenetic brain changes that map better onto genetic risk and, as a result, perform better in predicting treatment and prognosis than current approaches. However, thus far, this approach has not delivered strong find-ings upon which to revise diagnostic practices. Unless genetically valid subtypes are defined, shared liability adds a constraint on the future use of RPS to discriminate between psychiatric diagnoses as opposed to the less challenging, or less useful, distinction between those who do and do not have a major psychiatric syndrome.The remaining known schizophrenia risk loci are copy number variant (CNV) deletions or duplications of DNA segments from a thousand to a few million bases. CNVs have relatively large effects on risk with odds ratios of between 2 and 60, although, because they are rare, individual CNVs do not contribute substantially to the overall population risk of schizophrenia. Even for individual carriers, the diagnostic value of these CNVs with respect to schizo-phrenia is limited, with 2–20% of carriers depending on the CNV developing the disorder. However, all known schizophrenia associated CNVs are pleiotropic and contribute to a range of other disorders, including intellectual disability, autism spectrum disorder, ADHD, epilepsy and congenital malformations. The proportion of carriers who develop one or more of the above conditions is very high (approximately 50%) and for some loci is even higher.For those already affected with schizophrenia, knowl-edge of CNV carrier status might be relevant mainly for its explanatory power as people have a strong desire for an explanation of their condition but also because several CNVs are associated with high risks of comorbid medical phenotypes that might be overlooked in people with psychosis who often do not gain access to general health care. Owing to the high risk of developmental disorder for the offspring of these carriers, there is a case for making pathogenetic CNV testing available for patients with schizophrenia, of whom 2.5–8% are estimated to be carriers. Other classes of rare mutation play a part in schizophrenia, but early indications suggest that their overall contribution might be much lower than for common variation, which limits their role in general prediction and diagnostics. However, evidence supports the notion that deleterious point mutations in a subset of genes act analogously to CNVs in terms of effect size and pleiotropic effects, suggesting that when relevant mutations are identified, similar arguments for the screening of affected individuals might be applicable.At present, with the exception of the small number of known pathogenetic CNVs that we consider to be of possible clinical use, genetic findings might be useful in a research setting but do not provide the high precision that is re□uired for diagnosis or accurate risk prediction. Indeed, it is unlikely that genetics alone will ever achieve this goal. However, as more of the genetic variance that underlies schizophrenia is captured, risk profile scores derived from common, and possibly rare, genetic variation could plausibly contribute to risk algorithms. Undoubtedly, those algorithms will need to incorpor-ate additional indicators of risk, such as family history, environ mental variables (for example, drug use and severe childhood adversity) and developmental m arkers that either index risk or are themselves early markers of the disorder (for example, developmental delay, neurological soft signs minor abnormalities in sensory and motor performance identified by clinical examination and educational failure). Developing these algor-ithms will require much better research that is aimed at determining whether these indicators add to genetic risk, are non independent manifestations of genetic risk (for example, family history) or are even perhaps mediators of that risk (for instance, drug use). Moreover, even if prediction becomes possible, the benefits of implementation and the reᵁuired degree of specificity and sensitivity are crucially linked to the availability of interventions that can prevent or ameliorate the course of the disorder.

Can a Person Recover from Schizophrenia?

If a person with Schizophrenia gets the right treatment and the support they need, they can manage their symptoms. Many people can lead full lives, even if they still have symptoms or relapses from time to time. While there is currently no cure for schizophrenia, it can be treated effectively with medication and psychological treatment. It is not possible to predict how schizophrenia will affect someone's life, because the symptoms, severity and pattern of illness over time differ widely between

people. The impact of the illness also depends on the treatment and support they get to recover and stay well.The risk of being unable to work or live independently is higher when schizophrenia remains untreated for a long time or when a person does not get support to continue friendships and normal activities.

About one in seven people with schizophrenia recover almost completely. Some people with schizophrenia only ever have one episode of psychosis and then recover well. Many have more than one episode, with good recovery or at least some recovery

after each episode.

Other health problems for people with schizophrenia

People with schizophrenia often have other problems with their mental health and physical health. These can include:

- anxiety and depression
- problems with drug and alcohol use
- health problems caused by smoking
- physical health problems.

People with schizophrenia have high rates of smoking and many use other drugs of addiction. This may be part of the illness. Treatment for schizophrenia helps people deal with these problems. People with schizophrenia often neglect their physical health because they (and the people around them) tend to concentrate on their mental health problems. They need support and encouragement to stay healthy and avoid preventable illnesses like heart disease and diabetes.

Suicide is one of the main causes of death for people with schizophrenia. This is mainly because they can experience severe depression, especially in the early stages of the illness. Treatment aims to overcome depression and keep the person safe.

What Treatment is Available?

The most effective treatment for schizophrenia involves medication, psychological therapy and support with managing its impact on everyday life. Education about the illness and learning to respond effectively to the early warning signs of an episode are important. The development of anti-psychosis medications has revolutionised the treatment of schizophrenia. Now, most people can live in the community rather than be hospitalised. Some people are never hospitalised and their health care is delivered entirely in the community. Medications work by correcting the chemical imbalance in the brain associated with the illness. Newer, but well tested, medications promote a more complete recovery and have fewer side effects.

Schizophrenia is an illness, like many physical illnesses. Just as insulin is a lifeline for a person with diabetes, antipsychosis medications can be a lifeline for a person with schizophrenia. As with diabetes, some people will need to take medication indefinitely to keep symptoms under controland prevent recurrent episodes of psychosis.

Lifestyle changes, such as reducing harmful alcohol and other drug use and other triggers of episodes, can assist people to recover. Although there is no known cure for

schizophrenia, regular contact with a doctor or psychiatrist and possibly a multidisciplinary team (that might comprise mental health nurses, social workers, occupational therapists and psychologists) can help people to manage their symptoms and live full and productive lives. Peer support can also be a valuable source of support, useful information and hope. Sometimes, specific therapies directed towards symptoms, such as delusions, can be helpful. Physical health problems also need to be attended to.

Psychiatric disability rehabilitation services and support can help with problems related

to work, finances, accommodation, social relationships and loneliness. The family and friends of people with schizophrenia can often feel confused and distressed. Support and education, as well as better community understanding, are an important part of treatment.

Environment Contributes to Schizophrenia

It is very much important to understand that whenever the researchers use the term "environment", they generally talk about a broad definition. This definition includes everything but not the genetic factors or "genes". For a common person, environment signifies the house or the surrounding area or the neighborhood. The scientists are trying to evaluate the factors which are responsible for influencing the development of schizophrenia. For the scientists, the term environment includes every aspect from chemical, hormonal, nutritional and social environment during the pregnancy period. All the factors that affect the baby in the womb of the mother are well-studied.

These factors may result in social dynamics and may also stress the baby in latter life. Generally the problems can arise from drug use, use of different vitamins, education, and virus exposure and so much more. The causes of schizophrenia are wide and quite complex. It is basically the similar as "nature vs. nurture". We call it as "genes vs. environment" in finding the environment causes of schizophrenia. Even a single mistake or problem in environment may also contribute to the development of this mental disorder. It needs a great deal of study and in-depth research.

Several studies say that a child born during the winter season (January to March) in the Northern hemisphere has over 10% higher risk of schizophrenia. On the other side, an individual born in an urban environment is at 50% risk of developing schizophrenia. Another important study says that if the mother of the child has Rubella, the child has a 500% increased risk of schizophrenia. Flu and maternal infections during pregnancy are also related to the development of this mental disorder. This point of view has been given a wider level of response. Several psychologists agree to this point of view.

When the environmental factors come along with the genetic factors, there is an increase in the risk of getting diagnosed with schizophrenia. Birth location and economics is another factor. It has been found that people who are born in poverty are at higher risk of the mental health disorders. Moreover, in the urban environments, nutritional deficits and poverty may exist. The environmental factors can not be ignored. They are of utmost importance when schizophrenia is studied. It is essential to treat this mental disorder on time to avoid any kind of violent behaviors. An expert clinical psychologist is the best man to treat the problem with perfection.

Can We Cure Schizophrenia in the Next Decade?

Is it possible to cure schizophrenia? Well, many of the students graduating today with Psychiatric Degrees believe it is possible and they are primed to do it. Indeed curing Schizophrenia would be an incredible gift to humanity.

Most people do not realize just how prevalent this is in our society. I often wonder if this has anything to do with all the "Cults" which spring up. I have often wondered if completely curing Schizophrenia is a good idea because it is widely believed that those with even mild schizophrenia have a greater IQ than the average person in the population by 15 pts. Ever think of that?

If Schizophrenia were cured would that mean that our society would have less "high-intellegent" people in it? Could our society survive in that case if a percentage of the high-IQ people were removed due to a cure in Schizophrenia? Obviously those with severe Schizophrenia need help. But those who have mild Schizophrenia seem to function and you meet them every once in a while in society.

What are the statistics of those with schizophrenia? About 1-2 per hundred or something like that have schizophrenia and that does seem to be ⬜uite high. What are your thoughts on the impact on this? What about Religion, as if you stop schizophrenia then will religion disappear? Will the number of followers drop off?.

This is not to say that those who are religious are schizophrenic, but if they are hearing voices in their heads or talking to invisible friends then there are some psychological issues that probably should be addressed. Something to think on.

Treatment of Schizophrenia

Effective treatment can help you:

> overcome psychotic symptoms (e.g. delusions, hallucinations)

> get back in control of your thoughts, emotions and behaviours

> get back to school, study or work

> keep your friendships and social life stay healthy

How is Schizophrenia Treated?

The best treatment for schizophrenia is a combination of medication, psychological treatment and community support.

To plan your treatment, your health care team need to know all about your situation. As well as checking your symptoms and physical health, they will need to understand about your home, finances, and social life.

When should treatment start?

Getting help as soon as possible gives you the best chance of a good recovery, at any stage, including:

- at the first signs of ongoing emotional distress or significant changes in behaviour (e.g. becoming socially withdrawn, thinking about suicide or attempting suicide)
- a first episode of psychosis if you have hallucinations or delusions, even if you have never had psychosis before
- during a relapse when symptoms come back after you have been treated for schizophrenia.

A schizophrenia patient will most likely exhibit these signs:

- Becoming a recluse
- Hostility or suspiciousness
- Lackadaisical or careless in maintaining personal hygiene
- Staid but expressionless gaze
- Inability to cry or express joy
- Bizarre laughter or crying
- Depression
- Sleeplessness or oversleeping
- Odd or irrational statements
- Forgetful, unable to concentrate
- Hyper to criticism
- Strange usage of words or way of speaking

When a family member exhibits any of the above symptoms, it is advisable to consult a treatment center at the earliest.

A recent study claims that schizophrenia comprises eight distinct genetic disorders, all of which exhibit their own specific symptoms. The researchers claim that their findings would immensely help in diagnosis and treatment of the disease.

It was discovered that genetics play a huge role in determining the course of the disorder in a particular patient. People with relatives suffering from schizophrenia are somewhat predisposed to get the disease. Approximately 1 percent of the population in the U.S. has schizophrenia, but 10 percent of such patients have a first-degree relative with the disorder, which is a clear indication of a genetic predisposition to get the disease.

Tips to Lower Risk of Schizophrenia in Children

Ignoring the symptoms of schizophrenia and leaving it untreated can lead to severe complications. It is a mental disorder that affects a person's behavior and the way he feels and thinks. A schizophrenic loses touch with reality.

Schizophrenia runs in the genes, but it is not necessary that everyone in the family of an affected person would inherit the disease. It only increases the probability of its occurrence. Almost 85 percent people do not inherit schizophrenia despite having someone in the family suffering from it, while there are also those who get it even when there is no family history.

Reasons other than Genetics

Besides genetics, there are other reasons that can trigger schizophrenia in an individual:

Pregnancy complications, traumatic experiences in childhood such as sexual abuse, psychological abuse, and brain injury are also contributing factors that could lead to schizophrenia.

Abusing illicit drugs at an early age also precipitates the onset of the disease.

Any discordant and strained relationship with family members is also said to be a major reason for schizophrenia.

Environment and life situations also hasten the development of the disorder in an individual. A poor person is more vulnerable to get the disease than a prosperous one.

Incidentally, there are also reports which predict high occurrences of schizophrenia in rich countries as well. Seeking the best of treatments like the schizophrenia treatment can be a viable option for patients. The schizophrenia disorder treatment is counted among the best in the country.

However, when there is a family history of schizophrenia, certain precautions become necessary to prevent or lessen the effects of schizophrenia for the rest, especially the children. Because landing up in a schizophrenia treatment center cannot be a desirable situation for anybody, even if it is the reputed schizophrenia treatment.

Following are a few tips that would help in keeping the children safe from getting the disease:

Extending love and support to children: If there is a family history of schizophrenia, children in such households should be treated with utmost love and care. Any confrontation, abuse of mental, physical and emotional should be avoided at all cost. Such harsh behavior of parents and elders could trigger symptoms of schizophrenia in them.

Forging friendly relationship with kids: A friendly relationship with the children and helping them make friends outside can prevent them from feeling isolated. It will boost their self-esteem and thwart the advancement of schizophrenia signs. It is especially true of teenagers in the family.

Keeping kids occupied: The children should be encouraged to involve more into activities, like art and crafts, sports, music or other activities. Engagement will help them enhance their cognitive and emotional ‍uotients.

Teaching them to manage stress: Handing out lessons to children on how to manage stress will go a long way. Coping with stress can really help keep schizophrenia at bay. These learned skills will hold them in good stead later in life.

Nurturing their physical health: Right from choosing a healthy diet rich in nutrients to encouraging adequate physical activity, and nurturing a good physical health in the children will act as a deterrence to the onset of schizophrenia. They should be shielded and protected from getting any head injuries.

Giving them foods rich in omega-3 fatty acids: Researches have found that omega-3 fatty acids, or fish oil, may decrease the risk of psychotic disorders. Children should be given enough fishes like salmon, tuna, herrings and mackerel as they are rich in omega-3 fatty acids. Vegetarians can try flax seeds which are a good source of omega-3 fatty acids.

Specialised Programs for First Episode Psychosis

If you or someone you care for is experiencing a first episode of psychosis, it is important to get specialised care as soon as possible. Ask your doctor what special programs or services for people with first episode psychosis are available in your area. A private psychiatrist or a self-help group may also be able to help you get into a suitable program.

Medication for Schizophrenia

Most people with schizophrenia will need medication as part of their treatment. Medication works best when it is combined with psychological treatment. Antipsychotic medications (also called antipsychotics) are the main type of medication used to treat schizophrenia. Examples of antipsychotic medications are amisulpride, olanzapine, ☐uetiapine and risperidone. There are several different brand names for most of these medications. Clozapine is another antipsychotic medication, which is used to treat people who haven't had good results from other medications.

When you are starting any new medication, your doctor should explain the expected benefits. They should also explain the possible side effects, and make sure you understand.

Facts about medications for Schizophrenia

> ➤ Antipsychotic medications work well for managing hallucinations and delusions.
> ➤ Antipsychotic medications may also be helpful for anxiety and agitation, and problems with mood, thinking and socialising.
> ➤ Taking antipsychotic medication will not change your personality.
> ➤ Most people will only need to take one medication, but some people may need several.
> ➤ Most antipsychotic medications are tablets, capsules or li☐uid taken every day.

> Some antipsychotic medications are available as an injection. You would go to a clinic each week or month for an injection by a doctor or nurse.

> Antipsychotic medications are not addictive.

How long will I have to keep taking Medication?

How long you need to take antipsychotic medication for depends on your symptoms. Some people need to keep taking it long term. If you have only had one psychotic episode and you have recovered well, you would normally need to continue treatment for 1–2 years after recovery. If you have another psychotic episode, you may need to take antipsychotic medication for longer, up to five years. This is because the risk of schizophrenia symptoms recurring (relapse) is high for the first few years after a psychotic episode.

People who have had several psychotic episodes may need to keep taking antipsychotic medication for most of their life. Getting the most out of your schizophrenia medication

> Take every dose of your medication at the time recommended by your psychiatrist.

> When starting an antipsychotic medication, give it time to start working properly.

> Never stop or change your medication unless you and your psychiatrist talk about it and agree to change your treatment plan.

> If you have symptoms that you think could be side effects of medications, tell your doctor as soon as possible.

> It can take time to find the right type and dose of medication to manage your symptoms. Work with your doctor to find what works best for you.

> When you take an antipsychotic medication, your doctor should check your weight and do blood tests for diabetes and cholesterol levels. These checks should be done when you start taking the medication, several times during the first year, then once each year after that.

> If you take clozapine you need to be in a special program for regular health checks.

What are the Side Effects?

Antipsychotic medications can sometimes cause side effects. Side effects differ between antipsychotic medications and between people. Ask your doctor or pharmacist to explain the possible side effects, and ask for a printed leaflet. If you have side effects that bother you, speak to your doctor about them. They might be able to reduce the side effects by changing the dose of medication or switching to a different medication. Some side effects can be treated with other medications.

Side effects can include:

> weight gain. This is more common with olanzapine or clozapine. Putting on too much

> weight can increase your risk of other health problems, such as diabetes or heart disease. Some people can control their weight gain by healthy eating and physical activity. Other people need extra help or a change of medication. Your doctor might be able to refer you to a dietitian or weight management clinic.

> *Schizophrenia Your Health in Mind*

- drowsiness, sleepiness. This is more common with ꪛuetiapine, olanzapine and clozapine. This can be less of a problem if the medication is taken at night.

- constipation. If constipation is not severe, it can be managed by drinking more water, eating plenty of foods that are rich in fibre, and occasional use of mild laxatives.

- increased levels of blood fats and sugars, and high blood pressure. This is more common with medications that cause weight gain. Your GP can do regular check-ups to catch these problems early, so they can be treated.

- breast problems. Problems can include breast swelling or unusual secretion of breast milk.

- sexual problems. For example, problems getting aroused, or problems with erections and ejaculation. Speak to your doctor about these important side effects there are ways of managing them.

- dizziness or light-headedness. This is more common with sedating antipsychotic medications (e.g. chlorpromazine, clozapine). These problems normally happen after getting up from lying down or sitting.

- problems with nerves and muscles. These problems can include trembling, muscle stiffness, muscle spasm, tremor, slowed-down movement, restlessness, or a feeling of being unable to sit still.

- dry mouth.

What if the medication doesn't work for me? If you have tried one or two antipsychotic medications and your symptoms have not improved, you will need a thorough review.

First, your doctor will check that you have remembered to take the medication regularly, check that the dose was correct, and check for other possible causes, such as medical problems or cannabis use.

- ➤ Your doctor may suggest other treatments, such as:
- ➤ psychological treatment
- ➤ adding another medication
- ➤ trying a depot (injection) medication
- ➤ switching to clozapine.

Clozapine sometimes works when other medications have not. If you need to take clozapine, you will need regular check-ups, including blood tests.

Taking antipsychotic medication every day

Many people with schizophrenia find it hard to keep taking their medications. If you have trouble remembering to take your medication, or you are taking several different medications, ask your pharmacist to package your tablets in containers with compartments for each day. They might use a blister pack (sometimes called a Webster-Pak or Medico Pak) or a plastic container (called a dosette box). You may decide that a depot injection would be best for you. It is a good idea to always go to the same pharmacy so they can keep track of all your medications and give advice about them when needed.

Can I be forced to take my Medication?

You can be given treatment without your consent if you are at risk of harming yourself or others. This is called involuntary treatment. If the risks are very severe you may have to spend time in hospital while you receive treatment. If this happens, your doctor should give you a booklet that explains your rights. If you don't get a booklet, ask for it.

Involuntary treatment can only continue while it is necessary to keep you safe. You, and your family or carers, have the right to have the decision reviewed by an independent authority, such as a court or tribunal.

Pregnancy and Breastfeeding

For many antipsychotic medications, we don't yet know if they're safe for pregnant women to take. Some medications could harm an unborn baby, but stopping antipsychotic medication during pregnancy is risky for the mother. If you are planning to get pregnant, discuss this with your doctor. It's best if you plan how to keep yourself

and your baby safe before you get pregnant. If you are already pregnant, talk to your doctor as soon as possible about keeping yourself and your baby safe during pregnancy and breastfeeding.

Other medication

As well as your antipsychotic medication, your GP or psychiatrist may prescribe other medications to manage your symptoms.

Common examples include:

> anti-anxiety medications

- ➤ anti-depressant medications
- ➤ medications to manage abnormal mood changes, such as lithium, carbamazepine or sodium valproate (mood stabilisers)
- ➤ sleeping tablets
- ➤ medications to treat the side effects of antipsychotic medications.

It is also a good idea to take fish oil supplements ask your pharmacist which is the best one.

Psychological Treatment

Psychological Treatment (talking Therapy) helps you live with schizophrenia and have the best possible quality of life. For psychological treatment to work well, you need a good working relationship with your doctor or other therapist. You need to be able to trust them and stay hopeful about your recovery.

Types of Psychological Treatment for Schizophrenia include cognitive behavioural therapy (usually called CBT), psychoeducation and family psychoeducation.

Cognitive behavioural therapy (CBT) CBT is a type of psychological treatment that can help you:

- ➤ feel less distressed about your psychotic experiences
- ➤ feel less depressed and anxious
- ➤ reduce alcohol and drug use
- ➤ deal with suicidal thoughts
- ➤ overcome feelings of hopelessness.
- ➤

Cognitive Remediation

If you find you have problems with thinking, there are programs that can help. Cognitive remediation programs can help you improve your attention, memory and organisation skills. There are also programs that help you work on the way you interact with other people.

Psychoeducation

Psychoeducation helps people with schizophrenia (and their partner or family) understand the illness. Psychoeducation programs explain about symptoms, treatment options, recovery, and services that can help. You can have psychoeducation individually or in groups. It can include written information, videos, websites, meetings, or discussions with your case manager or psychiatrist.

Your family can help you understand your diagnosis and support you in your treatment. Family psychoeducation programs help the person with schizophrenia and their family communicate better and solve problems. Family psychoeducation is also good for family members. It can be very upsetting to see someone you love become unwell with schizophrenia.

Self-Care for Schizophrenia

Try to have a good relationship with the professionals involved in your care. Be honest and open. This will make it easier for them to understand and help you. When you and your doctor have found the medication and dose that works best for you, keep taking it don't skip doses or give up. Learn to recognise the signs that you could be having a relapse. Pay attention to changes in your body and in your thinking. Tell your mental health team or psychiatrist as soon as possible if you think something is going wrong.

Ask your case manager or psychiatrist to help you make a plan about how to deal with early signs of relapse. You can ask your close friends and family to help you if this happens. It is very important that you attend all of your appointments. You will need to have health checkups and screening tests to help you look after your physical health.

Keep in touch with your friends. Nurture all the positive relationships in your life. Be optimistic about your future. You can live with schizophrenia, and live well as you recover.

Looking after your body

- Try to keep up healthy eating habits and do regular physical exercise. Your health care team can give you advice on how to do this.
- If you smoke, try to stop. Smoking can interfere with your medications and stop them working properly. There are a range of programs to help people □uit, so ask your doctor or case manager about what is available in your local area. Usually people need many attempts before they finally □uit, so keep trying.

- If you use alcohol, drink sensibly. Heavy drinking makes living with schizophrenia even harder. It can make it hard to remember to take your medication and look after your physical health.
- Avoid illegal drugs. Heavy cannabis use can affect your recovery. It can also lead to relapse. Stimulant drugs like methamphetamine (including 'ice') or cocaine can trigger a psychotic episode and make symptoms worse.
- Don't have too much caffeine.
- Get regular sleep.
- Learn stress management techniques. If you have a case manager they may be able to help, or your GP can refer you to a psychologist to help with this.

Help with work or study

People with schizophrenia can find it hard to stay in paid work. It can be very hard to look after yourself and meet employers' expectations at the same time.

Programs may be available to help you get back into work or study. These could include training for work, or work programs (supported employment).

Supported employment programs are very successful in helping people get and keep a job. These programs can help you find a suitable job or course of study, and then help you keep working. Ask your case manager or psychiatrist if a program is available near where you live.

Coping with bad times

Suicidal thinking is usually only temporary, but it is dangerous to try to cope with it on your own.

Your treatment plan should include information about who to call if you need help, including when your normal doctors are not available

Public mental health crisis assessment teams (sometimes called CAT teams) are trained mental health professionals linked to your local health service. In a crisis, you can call them to speak about your situation, treatment and symptoms.

If necessary, they can visit you or arrange followup with your own treatment team. Ask your case manager for the phone number, and make sure you have it with you.

Help with Living Arrangements

Many people with schizophrenia have problems finding and keeping a suitable place to live. Local services and support organisations can help ask your health care team or support worker for more information.

Help with Social Skills

Social rehabilitation programs can help you get back to mixing comfortably with other people. Ask your case manager or psychiatrist if a program is available near where you live.

Social skills training: Patients with schizophrenia may need to re-learn how to appropriately interact in social situations. This kind of psychosocial intervention involves rehearsing or role-playing real-life situations so the person is prepared when they occur. This type of training can reduce drug use, and improve relationships.

Group Activities

If you are living with schizophrenia, it can help to take part in group activities. It is harder and slower to recover when you are lonely. People in groups can benefit from each other's experiences. They are also an opportunity to make new friends. The friendly support you get from your group reminds you that you are not alone – other people have mental illnesses and are coping with many of the same problems as you.

Mental health workers or local community groups sometimes organise group activities for people with mental illness. These activities could help you:

> - get reliable information
> - earn how to cope with your mental illness
> - be more active and keep fit
> - make friends
> - become more independent
> - become more confident
> - cope with problems
> - with your study or work
> - have fun
> - feel less alone by sharing experiences with people who are also living with mental health issues. Ask your case manager or psychiatrist if group activities are available near where you live.

Counselling

Talking to someone is an important part of treatment.

Your case manager and psychiatrist can provide general counselling and support during and after an episode of psychosis

Mood swings and depression are common in patients with schizophrenia. In addition to antipsychotics, other types of medications are used.

Mood stabilizers include:

- ➢ lithium (Lithobid)
- ➢ divalproex (Depakote)
- ➢ carbamazepine (Tegretol)
- ➢ lamotrigine (Lamictal)
- ➢ Antidepressants include:
- ➢ fluoxetine (Prozac)
- ➢ sertraline (Zoloft)
- ➢ paroxetine (Paxil)
- ➢ citalopram (Celexa)
- ➢ escitalopram (Lexapro)
- ➢ venlafaxine (Effexor)
- ➢ desvenlafaxine (Pristiq)
- ➢ duloxetine (Cymbalta)
- ➢ bupropion (Wellbutrin)

Family psycho-education teaches family members problem-solving skills.

Schizophrenia Treatment - Psychosocial Interventions

Family psychoeducation: It is important to include psychosocial interventions in the treatment of schizophrenia. Including family members to support patients decreases the relapse rate of psychotic episodes and improves the person's outcomes. Family relationships are improved when everyone knows how to support their loved one dealing with schizophrenia. A psychiatrist, nurse, case manager, employment counselor, and substance-abuse counselor often make up an ACT team.

Assertive Community Treatment (ACT): Another form of psychosocial intervention includes use of out-patient support groups. Support teams including psychiatrists, nurses, case managers, and other counselors, meet regularly with the schizophrenic patient to help reduce the need for hospitalization or a decline in their mental status.

About 50% of individuals with schizophrenia suffer from some kind of substance abuse or dependence.

Substance abuse treatment: Many people with schizophrenia (up to 50%) also have substance abuse issues. These substance abuse issues worsen the behavioral symptoms of schizophrenia and need to be addressed for better outcomes.

A group socializes around a laptop computer.

Supported employment: Many people with schizophrenia have difficulty entering or reentering the work force due to their condition. This type of psychosocial intervention helps people with schizophrenia to construct resumes, interview for jobs, and even connects them with employers willing to hire people with mental illness.

A doctor uses cognitive behavioral therapy (CBT) intervention with a patient.

Cognitive Behavioral Therapy (CBT): This type of intervention can help patients with schizophrenia change disruptive or destructive thought patterns, and enable them to function more optimally. It can help patients "test" the reality of their thoughts to identify hallucinations or "voices" and ignore them. This type of therapy may not work in actively psychotic patients, but it can help others who may have residual symptoms that medication does not alleviate.

Weight gain can be a side effect of some antipsychotic and other psychiatric medications.

Weight management: Many antipsychotic and psychiatric drugs cause weight gain as a side effect. Maintaining a healthy weight, eating a well-balanced diet, and exercising regularly helps prevent or alleviate other medical issues. A family supports each other.

What Is the Prognosis for Schizophrenia?

The prognosis for people with schizophrenia can vary depending on the amount of support and treatment the patients receives. Many people with schizophrenia are able to function well and lead normal lives. However, people with schizophrenia have a higher death rate and higher incidence of substance abuse. When medications are taken regularly and the family is supportive, patients can have better outcomes.

Treatment phases and goals Treatment of schizophrenia targets various domains, including positive symptoms, agitation and aggres-sion, negative symptoms, cognitive dysfunction, mood symptoms, suicidality, QOL, and social, academic and vocational functioning. Accordingly, management goals include reduction of acute symptoms, 'response', which is defined as the reduction of total symptoms compared with baseline by at least 20% (that is, at least minimally improved) to 40–50% (that is, at least much improved), and remission, which is defined as only mild positive and negative symptoms sustained for at least most of these findings are based on individual hence unreplicated studies in small samples of patients. By contrast, more-consistent evidence has been produced with clinical predictors of poor antipsychotic response, such as male sex, younger age at disease onset, longer duration of untreated illness, poor premorbid adjust-ment, severe baseline psychopathology, non-adherence to antipsychotics, co-morbidities (especially substance use disorders), a lack of early minimal antipsychotic response and longer illness duration or non-first-episode illness. Moreover, emerging evidence suggests that, after each relapse, a certain percentage of patients do not respond as well to the same or different antipsychotics as they did originally. Conversely, a lack of improvement with nonclozapine antipsychotics predicts clozapine response. Furthermore, although therapeutic blood monitoring of antipsychotic concentrations has been proposed in the past, current established thresholds only exist for clozapine, for which a minimum level of 350–450 ng per dl is thought to be needed for robust clozapine response.

Conse☐uences of Schizophrenia

Mortality

Although schizophrenia is not in itself a fatal disease, death rates of people with schizophrenia are at least twice as high as those in the general population. The excess mortality has been related in the past to poor conditions of prolonged institutional care, leading to high occurrence of tuberculosis and other communicable diseases. This may still be an important problem wherever large numbers of patients spend a long time in crowded asylum like institutions.

However, recent studies of people with schizophrenia living in the community showed suicide and other accidents as leading causes of death in both developing and developed countries. Suicide, particularly, has emerged as a growing matter of concern, since lifetime risk of suicide in schizophrenic disorders has been estimated at above 10%, which is about 12 times that of the general population. There seems to be an increased mortality for cardiovascular disorders as well, possibly related to unhealthy lifestyles, restricted access to health care or the side effects of antipsychotic drugs.

Social Disability

According to the International classification of impairments, disability and handicaps impairment represents any loss or abnormality of psychological, physiological or anatomical structure or function, while disability is any restriction or lack (resulting from an impairment) of ability to perform an activity in the manner or within the range considered normal for an individual in his or her socio cultural setting.

In mental disorders, such as schizophrenia, disability can affect social functioning in various broad areas, namely:

> - self care, which refers to personal hygiene, dressing and feeding;
> - occupational performance, which refers to expected functioning in paid activities, studying, homemaking;
> - functioning in relation to family and household members, which refers to expected interactions with spouses, parents, children or other relatives;

> functioning in a broader social context, which refers to socially appropriate interaction with community members, and participation in leisure and other social activities.

Data from European and North American studies show persisting disability of moderate or severe degree in about 40% of males with schizophrenia, in contrast with 25% of females. Substantially lower figures have been found in India, Africa and Latin America. Global assessment of disability, however, hides wide variations across life domains, which can be affected in different ways. There is good evidence that for most patients nature and extent of social disability are more relevant as outcome indicators than clinical symptoms.

Social Stigma

Social stigma refers to a set of deeply discrediting attributes, related to negative attitudes and beliefs towards a group of people, likely to affect a person's identity and thus leading to a damaged sense of self through social rejection, discrimination and social isolation. Stigma is strongly linked with the label of mentally ill and is, to a certain extent, unrelated to the actual characteristics or behaviours of those stigmatized. Various adverse conse uences may arise from the stigmatization process: use of pejorative language, barriers to housing or employment, restricted access to social services, fewer chances for marriage, increased mistreatment and institutionalization Stigma is deeply rooted in the cultural background of society. Some observers have pointed out that it is less pervasive in most rural societies, but this assumption has been challenged by cross-cultural studies. There is no convincing evidence that there are cultures in which stigma is not attached to major mental disorders, whatever theories people hold about their causes, although the process of negative labelling may concern different groups across cultures and the level of stigma may vary. Stigma operates however, not only in the larger community but within the mental health services as well. It may even be found at the level of the affected individuals as internalized negative self-perception .

Undoubtedly, stigma represents a major challenge with regard to the integration of persons with schizophrenia and other mental disorders into the community. Many first-person accounts from people with experience of mental disorder vividly portray the painful effects of stigmatization on their everyday lives.

Stigma also acts as a powerful barrier to treatment, not only because of the fear of being labelled as mentally ill, but also because too often mental health professionals and mental health services as a whole hold, often in a subtle way, negative or rejecting attitudes towards users and perpetuate practices fostering segregation, dependency and powerlessness.

Impact on Caregivers

The available data show that the proportion of persons with schizophrenia living with their relatives ranges between 40% in United States to more than 90% in China. Moreover, family involvement and distress is not necessarily lower when the sufferer lives away from home. Nevertheless, the burden that is often placed on families or others living in close contact with a mentally ill person has only recently been recognized. Various aspects of impact on caregivers should be considered, including:

> ➢ the economic burden related to the need to support the patient and the loss of productivity of the family unit;

> emotional reactions to the patient's illness, such as guilt, a feeling of loss and fear about the future;

> the stress of coping with disturbed behaviour;

> disruption of household routine;

> problems of coping with social withdrawal or awkward interpersonal behaviour;

> curtailment of social activities.

Various aspects of the caregiver's burden have been reported across a variety of geographical and social settings. Financial loss associated with schizophrenia has been noticed in different countries.

The manifold facets of burden hinder any overall evaluation, making it difficult to identify factors that are likely to influence it. A summary list includes patients' and caregivers' characteristics, family size and economic status, role expectations and illnessrelated beliefs. Such wide variability, combined with cross-cultural differences, leads to estimates of prevalence of family burden ranging between 30% and 80%. There is a widely held belief that distress is more often related to patients' apathy, inactivity or failure to comply with social duties, than with more evident positive psychotic symptoms or behavioural disturbances. However, this may not be true in all social or cultural groups. According to a recent survey in Malaysia, in which subjective emotional burden has been found in 41% of families, hostility, violence and disruption of family activities was perceived as the main source of stress.

Social Costs

In recent years a major effort has been made towards the ◻uantification of the global social burden of all illnesses and injuries, taking into account not only mortality but the extent of disability and allowing comparisons between Schizophrenia and public health different categories of illness. The measure of disability adjusted life years (DALYs) lost has been used as a health status indicator. Although this approach may not be completely suitable for most mental disorders, including schizophrenia, because of their variable course and the fluctuating nature of the related disability, it enables social scientists and policy-makers to put the burden associated with schizophrenia within a comprehensive public health framework. The loss in DALYs caused by schizophrenic disorders worldwide at slightly below 13 million, which represents about 1% of the global burden of the disease deriving from all causes. Schizophrenia is 26th in the list of the diseases, ranked according to their contribution to the overall burden.

However, if one takes into account the predicted modifications in social structure in most developing countries and the increase of populations at risk over the coming decades, schizophrenia is projected to be in 20th position by the year 2020, with more than 17 millions of DALYs lost, accounting for 1.25% of the overall burden. Estimates of economic costs of schizophrenia are available only for some industrialized countries. A broad distinction should be made between direct costs, i.e. money spent on providing care to affected individuals, and indirect costs, i.e. loss of resources and productivity due to morbidity and mortality. Direct costs of schizophrenia in western countries range between 1.6% and 2.6% of total health care expenditures, which in turn account for between 7% and 12% of the gross national product. This means £396 million in the United Kingdom and $18 billion in the United States (National Advisory Mental Health

Council). These costs, however, are very unevenly distributed among subgroups with differing severity of the disorder. According to a British study, if we consider a sample of people with schizophrenia from onset to death, it can be estimated that care of patients with long-term disabling course (which represent only 10% of the affected population) will absorb about 80% of the total lifetime direct costs. About 75% of these high costs are due to inpatient or residential care, while drugs represent less than 5%. Therefore, any strategy aimed at reducing the costs of care for schizophrenia should target the small group of most disabled patients in order to improve, as far as possible, their independent living skills.

Prevention, Treatment and Care

Preventive Interventions

Primary prevention refers to an intervention that is intended to reduce the incidence of an illness in a population which is as yet unaffected by the disease. Two broad primary preventive strategies can be used within a public health framework: illness prevention and health promotion. Illness prevention aims to establish specific interventions for specific disorders by modifying one or more risk factors, while health promotion aims to enhance health promoting behaviours in the community to maintain well-being and prevent the onset of broad groups of disorders.

Secondary prevention aims at early identification of individuals with prodromal or early symptoms of an illness to reduce morbidity through prompt treatment. A distinction between primary and secondary prevention depends on accurate knowledge of the natural history of the illness, with clear detection of prodromes, precursors and fullblown symptoms. At some point in time, when the onset of a disorder becomes inevitable, preventive strategies conceptually shift from primary to secondary. The complex multifaceted interplay that underlies the onset of schizophrenia, the low specificity of risk factors and prodromal symptoms, the lack of reliable methods to assess vulnerability to the disorder, and the uncertainties surrounding the pictures of its early course limit the development of targeted preventive interventions. Although the role of genetic transmission in liability to schizophrenia has been well documented, incomplete penetrance, the probable existence of non-genetic forms of the disorder and the absence of genetic markers make genetic risk prediction highly inaccurate. Moreover, only a small minority of people who develop schizophrenia come from families with a relative who is also affected. Such problems, in addition to ethical considerations, rule out the feasibility of genetic counselling.

It can be assumed that the prevention of obstetric complications, through the establishment of safer conditions for pregnancy and childbirth, could make a small contribution to the reduction of risk of schizophrenia, as well as of many other mental and neurological disorders. No data, however, are available to support this assumption.

Models for a psychosocial approach to the prevention of schizophrenia have recently been advocated.

They involve various combinations of the following strategies:

> community education programmes about psychoses;

> integration of mental health services in primary care;

> detection by general practitioners and other community agencies of early warning signs of severe mental disorder;

> intensive home-based assessment and interventions targeted at people at risk and key persons in their social networks to enhance stress management strategies and problem solving skills.

The underlying hypothesis is that the development of health promoting coping attitudes in people showing at-risk mental states and in their social environment could prevent the onset of overt schizophrenic disorders, even through non-specific interventions. Moreover, active treatment can be started quickly if frank psychosis occurs. Such approaches deserve attention insofar as they focus on the primary health care setting, thus reducing the stigma associated with psychiatric services and facilitating access to early treatment. All such aspects are particularly important, given that the treatment lag in first episode schizophrenia has been estimated at one year or even more. Their value as truly preventive strategies, however, remains so far uncertain. More research is needed in this area.

Drugs

The place of medications in the treatment of schizophrenia has been firmly established for some 40 years. Given the recent advances in psychopharmacology, it is useful to distinguish between conventional and atypical antipsychotic drugs.

Although their chemical structures vary widely, their common mode of action is to block dopamine D2 receptors mostly in mesolimbic and nigrostriatal brain areas. Their activity on psychotic symptoms is probably related to their action in the mesolimbic system. Although many are available, none has been shown to be more effective than any other, although for unknown reasons a particular patient may respond to one drug and be unimproved or even made worse by another. Evidence for their efficacy in reducing acute positive symptoms (not only in schizophrenia, but in any disorder with psychotic features) is clear-cut, while their impact on negative symptoms looks modest. Findings from a large number of clinical trials indicate a substantial improvement within 6-14 weeks in 75% of patients with acute symptoms of schizophrenia treated at a dosage of 300-750 mg of chlorpromazine equivalents, in comparison with less than 25% treated with placebo. Their efficacy in preventing relapse or recurrence after clinical remission, although well established, is less impressive. Risk of relapse during the first year following an acute episode in patients on antipsychotic medications is reduced to about 20%, in comparison with about 60% on placebo.

Data for more than one year are □uite limited and relapse rates on placebo and on medications may become similar after two or three years. Therefore, drug therapy delays but does not suppress relapses. There is no consensus on how long treatment should be continued following an acute episode. For first-episode patients, in case of full remission, it has been suggested that medication should be tapered or discontinued within six months to two years. For patients with multiple episodes or who show incomplete remission, there are no agreed guidelines; decisions about medication should be made on individual basis, balancing the costs and benefits of treatment. With respect to maintenance doses, concern about unnecessary exposure to high amounts of medication, resulting in risk of tardive dyskinesia and other side-effects, led to the development of methods for determining the lowest effective dose. Two approaches are the focus of interest: targeted and low dose strategies. So far, the use of low-dose strategy seems best supported by research. In fact, the benefits of such drugs in real practice are limited by a number of problems.

First of all, these drugs induce side-effects that are often distressing and sometimes dangerous. The most common are:

- sedation;
- extrapyramidal side-effects, such as tremors, acute dystonias, akathisia, akinesia, stiffness and shuffling gait;
- tardive dyskinesia;
- anticholinergic effects, such as dry mouth, blurred vision, urinary hesitancy, constipation;
- cardiovascular effects, such as tachycardia and postural hypotension;
- endocrine effects, such as amenorrhea, galactorrhea, breast enlargement in women and gynecomastia in men;
- weight gain;
- skin and eye effects, such as cutaneous rash, photo toxic skin reactions, pigmentary changes in skin, granular deposits in the cornea and lens;
- complication: It is an idiosyncratic reaction, presenting initially as muscular rigidity and neuroleptic malignant syndrome, which is a rare but serious and potentially fatal progressing to high fever, fluctuating consciousness and unstable vital signs.

Mortality has been reported in 20% of cases. Although most side-effects are mild and time-limited, some represent serious problems and deserve special attention. Akathisia and other extrapyramidal symptoms, occurring to some degree in up to 70% of patients, are associated with considerable subjective distress that includes restlessness, anxiety, irritability and inability to feel comfortable. Some reports suggest that severe akathisia can result in aggressive or suicidal acts. Tardive dyskinesia is a severe complication of long-term use of antipsychotics, characterized by a wide range of abnormal involuntary movements involving mouth, tongue, jaw or any other part of the body. Dyskinesia can be seriously disabling in its more severe forms and may affect walking, eating and breathing. Its incidence has been estimated at around 4% per year for 5-6 years of drug exposure and its prevalence in patients on maintenance treatment has been estimated to be at least 20%. The effects of extrapyramidal symptoms and abnormal movements go beyond their medical conse uences. According to research findings, strengthened by the personal accounts of patients, they may add to negative symptomatology even when unnoticed by clinicians and may impair, in more or less subtle ways, interpersonal skills. Treatment resistance is another relevant issue. Current data suggest that between 20-30% of patients fail to respond to acute treatment and the same proportion will relapse despite ade uate maintenance therapy.

Poor compliance with drug prescription is fairly common in the treatment of schizophrenia: about 50% of outpatients and 20% of inpatients fail to take prescribed medications. Even highly supervised settings and the use of depot injections cannot resolve the problem. Explanations offered for noncompliance centre on several areas: staff-patient conflict, adverse reactions to drugs and side- effects, lack of insight due to psychotic disorder, inadequate information on drugs, and the patients' negative view of medications.

Although any explanation, or combination of explanations, may be true for a single patient, the issue of compliance points to a major limitation of antipsychotics: the active refusal by a number of users to take medications and the unpleasant feelings and discomfort reported even by some who comply,

20 Nations for Mental Health willing or not, with treatment. Such problems, overlooked by most clinical trials, came only recently to the attention of researchers and clinicians. Health professionals should listen carefully to the subjective experience associated with medications to discuss in a collaborative way with users issues related to long-term drug treatment. In recent years great hopes have been raised by the introduction of so-called "new" or "atypical" antipsychotics, deemed free from most of the shortcomings of conventional ones. Atypical antipsychotics share two common features: action on mesolimbic neurons with little effect on nigrostriatal neurons, and higher 5-HT2 than D2 receptors affinity. This implies an effect on psychotic symptoms with a low incidence of extrapyramidal side-effects.

Clozapine is the first atypical antipsychotic to be introduced. It has been found to be as effective as antipsychotics on positive symptoms in both acute and maintenance treatment. Further, it has been found effective in improving psychotic symptoms in some 30-60% of schizophrenia patients who failed to respond to adeᨉuate dosage of conventional antipsychotics, and it is associated with a greatly reduced likelihood of developing extrapyramidal symptoms, neuroleptic malignant syndrome or tardive dyskinesia. However, clozapine produces other serious side-effects. It is associated with a risk of agranulocytosis of 1-2%, which is most likely to occur within the first six months of treatment. Because agranulocytosis can be fatal if not detected and reᨉuires immediate discontinuation of the drug, patients on clozapine must undergo monitoring of white blood cell count weekly for the first 18 weeks and subsequently every four weeks as long as they take the drug. Other unwanted effects include seizures in up to 10% of patients, weight gain, hypotension, tachycardia and sedation.

Clozapine is very expensive: the average annual cost per patient has been estimated at around £2000 in the United Kingdom and $8500 dollars in the USA, i.e. 10 or more times higher than the cost of standard drugs. Although preliminary studies suggest that clinical benefits may lead to medium-term cost savings, primarily by reducing hospitalization, more investigations are needed to clarify this important issue. Moreover, it should be remembered that cost-benefit analyses can hardly be generalized across social and health care systems. The need for regular blood sampling clearly limits the use of clozapine and may seriously affect patients' adherence to treatment, as shown by noncompliance rates of up to 50% found in some studies. The complexity of clozapine therapy seems at odds with the flexibility and easy access to treatment required by community care. Other atypical antipsychotics that are currently being marketed or developed include risperidone, olanzapine and quetiapine. New data indicates that these neuroleptic drugs are promising both from the point of view of efficacy and their side effect profile.

In summary, atypical antipsychotics represent the first innovation in biological treatment of psychoses in 40 years. However, many factors limit their widespread use at present. In the near future we shall see whether today's promises will be kept.

Family Interventions

The causal role of dysfunctional child-rearing patterns and disturbed family communication was a cornerstone of early social theories of schizophrenia. Such theories, although weakly supported by empirical data, enjoyed wide popularity among professionals, particularly in the USA and other western countries, unfortunately contributing to negative attitudes towards patients' relatives and adversarial relationships between professionals and families. Subsequent research moved away from ambitious causal explanations to identify, within the framework of studies of expressed emotion, factors related to family interaction and family members' beliefs and expectations that are likely to influence the course of schizophrenia, and other mental and physical disorders.

This approach resulted in the development of family-based interventions designed to enhance the resources of the family unit in its caring function, relieve family burden, and modify family interactions and affective attitudes predictive of relapse.

Such interventions, variously called "psychoeducational", "supportive" or "behavioural", share some common elements, namely:

> engagement of the family early in the treatment process in a "no fault" atmosphere;

> education about schizophrenia (the vulnerability-stress model, risk factors, variation in prognosis, rationale for various treatments, suggestions for coping with the disorder);

> communication training directed at enhancing the clarity of communication and improving the exchange of both positive and negative feedback within the family;

> problem solving training aimed at improving ways of managing everyday problems, coping with stressful life events, and planning to deal with anticipated stressors, by generalizing problem-solving skills;

> crisis intervention at times of extreme stress or when signs of relapse are evident.

A number of studies conducted in various geographical and cultural settings show that the inclusion of culturally sensitive family interventions in the comprehensive care of people with schizophrenia significantly reduces the risk of relapse and increases patients' and relatives' satisfaction with service. It is worth noting that some clinical trials supporting this evidence have been conducted in developing countries, such as China. In fact, in many cultures in Africa, Asia and Latin America families do represent the core community support system and family members have always been consideredprimary caregivers for their ill relatives. Therefore, collaboration between them and health professionals has been the rule and conflicting relationships have rarely developed.

The identification of family intervention as an important component of community care entails a conceptual and practical shift: family intervention should now be viewed, in most cases, as a long-term support rather than as a short time limited treatment.

Other Psychosocial Interventions

For several decades insight-oriented long-term psychodynamic psychotherapy, stemming from the psychoanalytic tradition, has been the mainstay, particularly in France, the USA and to a lesser extent other European countries, of the psychological approach to treatment of schizophrenia. The psychodynamic model enjoyed high status and heavily influenced the training and professional attitudes of many clinicians, although it has never been within easy reach for the average patient. Over the last 20 years disappointing results of carefully designed clinical trials, high costs and limited flexibility and adaptability to community settings, led to widespread dissatisfaction with exploratory psychodynamic psychotherapy. Attention shifted to a variety of other psychosocial interventions, deriving from cognitivebehavioural models or developed within the framework of psychosocial rehabilitation.

Direct treatment of cognitive functioning through structured psychological interventions has been recently introduced as a byproduct of neuropsychological studies of schizophrenia. The goal is to remedy problems of basic information-processing skills, such as memory, attention and conceptual abilities. So far, no consistent conclusion can be drawn about the efficacy of such an approach, which has to be considered in the early stages of development. Moreover, it is uncertain to what extent improvements in the basic domains of cognitive functioning, detected by neuropsychological tests, can affect more complex social performances. Another, perhaps more relevant, cognitive approach focuses on subjective response to dysfunctional thoughts or perceptions. It attempts to modify beliefs associated with delusions and ways of coping with auditory hallucinations. The strength of this model lies in its purpose, which is to build on natural coping strategies already used by people with schizophrenia when faced with positive symptoms, thus linking professional intervention with self-help efforts. Moreover, it emphasizes that psychotic symptoms lie on a continuum of differences in thought or behaviour and do not arise from fundamentally different psychological processes, challenging a long-held belief about the discontinuity between schizophrenia and ordinary experience. Preliminary results show that such techni ues have promise.

Other interventions are usually included under the heading of psychosocial rehabilitation and sometimes psychosocial rehabilitation itself is referred to as an intervention. This is misleading because psychosocial rehabilitation is not a techni ue, or a set of techni ues, but an overall strategy encompassing not only health services but also legislation, social policy and economy (WHO). It is more appropriate, therefore, to present such interventions, which are primarily addressed at the reduction of some aspects of disability and handicap associated with schizophrenia, as components of overall rehabilitation packages. Social skills training refers to a class of interventions, based on social learning theories, that aim to teach the perceptual, motor and interpersonal skills deemed relevant to achieving community survival, independence and socially rewarding relationships. Complex behaviours are assessed and broken down into smaller discrete components taught through various behavioural techniques such as problem specification, instruction, modelling, role playing, behavioural rehearsal, coaching, reinforcement, structured feedback and homework assignment. The focus of social skills training programmes has recently moved from topographical features of overt behaviour to a more comprehensive range of communication and independent living skills. There is little doubt that people with schizophrenia can learn a variety of social skills, ranging from simple motor behaviours to more complex ones such as assertiveness and conversational skills. The improvement is evident for specific behavioural performances but is less pronounced for interpersonal and daily living skills. However, it remains unclear whether such effects transfer from the training environment to everyday life. Furthermore, the impact of social skills training on aspects of patients' outcome has not yet been demonstrated. Changes in social skills training methods, including implementation in natural settings by utilization of cues and prompts in everyday life, are probably necessary to overcome such limitations. Vocational rehabilitation has a long history and has traditionally been provided through hospital or clinic-based workshop activities. However, the value of such an approach has been questioned on the basis of consistently negative data on patients' employment following discharge. A subsequent evolution of the field, i.e. sheltered employment programmes, also failed to show any impact on employment outside the sheltered environment.

Physical Health Premature Mortality

An important phenomenon observed among people with schizophrenia and other severe mental disorders is poor physical health and premature death. Such physical health disparities have rightfully been stated as contravening international conventions for the 'right to health'. The physical health of people with severe mental illness is commonly ignored not only by the service users themselves but also by people around them and even by health systems. People with severe mental disorders, including schizophrenia, experience disproportionately higher rates of mortality[6, 7], often due to physical illnesses such as cardiovascular diseases, metabolic diseases, and respiratory diseases . The mortality gap results in a 10-25 year life expectancy reduction in these patients. For people with schizophrenia, mortality rates are 2 to 2.5 times higher than the general population.

Physical Health Conditions

There is evidence to suggest that people with schizophrenia have higher prevalence rates of cardiovascular problems and obstetric complications (in women).

There is also good evidence that they are more likely to become overweight, develop diabetes, hyperlipidaemia, dental problems, impaired lung function, osteoporosis, altered pain sensitivity, sexual dysfunction and polydipsia or be affected by some infectious diseases such as HIV, hepatitis and tuberculosis as compared with the general population.

Unhealthy Life Style and Factors of Risk

Heavy smoking is about 2-6 times more prevalent among people with schizophrenia as compared with the general population, with prevalence rates between 50 and 80%. Even as compared with people with other severe mental illnesses, being a current smoker is 2-3 times more common among people with schizophrenia. Particularly high rates of smoking are observed among patients hospitalised for psychiatric treatment. Patients with schizophrenia are often at greater risk for being overweight or obese, with estimated prevalence rates between 45 and 55%. People with schizophrenia have demonstrated lower levels of physical activity and physical fitness than the general population, which may be due to the limited ability to be physically active, being overweight or obese, higher smoking rates and side effects from anti-psychotic medication.

Impact of Health and Treatment Systems

Institutionalization commonly robs service users of the space and the autonomy required for being mobile and physically active. Many institutions lack structured, balanced or individualised dietary regimes and people may gain weight and even become obese. Furthermore, many antipsychotic medicines increase appetite, and if not monitored regularly, may directly or indirectly contribute to substantial metabolic changes, which can lead to diabetes, hyperlipidaemia and hypertension. Estimated prevalence rates for diabetes and hypertension in patients with schizophrenia are between 10 and 15% and between 19 and 58% respectively. The elevated physical health risks associated with schizophrenia and other severe mental illnesses indicate a stronger need for close and regular health monitoring. Paradoxically, people with severe mental illness receive less medical care for their physical problems as compared with others. Being in good physical health is a crucial aspect for quality of life; however, it is known that people living with schizophrenia and other severe mental illnesses have a higher prevalence of physical diseases compared to the general population. Promoting collaboration between mental and physical health is vital for improving care of people with severe mental illness. The diagnosis of physical conditions is commonly overshadowed by a psychiatric diagnosis and delayed diagnosis makes interventions less effective or even impossible.

Mental and Social Health Problems

A common but harmful mistake is to identify people with schizophrenia simply as a clinical diagnosis. The inappropriate term "Schizophrenic" is commonly used by the public and even by some care givers to refer to a person who is living with schizophrenia. This term eclipses the human and social nature of that individual, and renders them as purely a diagnosis. People living with schizophrenia experience discrimination and violations of their rights both inside and outside institutions. In everyday life they face major problems in the areas of education, employment, and access to housing. As previously mentioned, even access to health services is more challenging. People living with a severe mental disorder are also likely to suffer from other mental disorders such as depression and substance abuse. Lifetime prevalence of suicide among those living with a severe mental disorder is around 5% which is much higher than that in the general population. Higher prevalence of substance use among people with schizophrenia along with some other factors contributes to the higher reported violent activity among them and to their higher rates of victimization alike.

People with severe mental illnesses, including schizophrenia are also more likely to be homeless, unemployed, or living in poverty.

Interventions

In many countries efforts have begun to better improve the physical health of people with schizophrenia, whilst simultaneously encouraging the social and education sector to provide better access to service for people with severe mental illness. Treatments should not be limited to pharmacotherapy. Non pharmacological psychosocial interventions are gaining an increasing importance and should be considered an adjunctive component of mental disorder management. Psychosocial interventions are also effective at preventing some of the side effects of antipsychotic medications. A meta-analysis has shown the enduring effects of a range of nonpharmacological interventions at reducing antipsychotic-induced weight gain, namely individual or group interventions, cognitive–behavioural therapy and nutritional counselling.

Living and Coping With Schizophrenia

Schizophrenia is a mental disorder which has no permanent cure. Its symptoms can be dormant in one moment while severely aggravated in other moments, depending on the effectiveness of the medications and treatments the Schizophrenic patient is taking. Schizophrenia is very detrimental as it takes away loved ones, family, friends and sometimes one's ability to make a living. In order to live life again, it is important for Schizophrenic patients to learn how to cope this dreadful disorder. Following are some of the suggestions which can be used for coping and living with Schizophrenia.

Acceptance of the Reality

The patient must admit the fact that he is suffering from Schizophrenia. Usually, a Schizophrenic patient denies his suffering. He thinks that people are lying to him; this is because of basic human tendency of refusal to things which prove one wrong. As the same time, Schizophrenia patient suffer from hallucinations which make it extremely challenging for him to differentiate between real life and illusion. To handle this situation, families must lend their supporting hand to manage his medication taking and making sure he attends his psychotherapy session. The patient should also be sent for group therapy where he is made to realize that if he admits that he is suffering from the mental illness, it will make his life and others around him far easier. The patient who has admitted to reality is more likely to take his medications on time, discuss openly during psychotherapy sessions and gain the most out of all his treatments.

Knowledge about Schizophrenia

Knowledge about Schizophrenia is no doubt very important in order to cope with it. Patient with Schizophrenia will be in a better position to cope with the illness if they fully understand it. Family members will also be more understanding of the situation and response better to the patient. Hence, it is vastly important for the patient and family members to learn about the symptoms associated with Schizophrenia.

Living Independently in a Safe Neighborhood

A Schizophrenic patient whose family members refuse to take care of him either due to lack of understanding or lack of funds can possibly live in an independent setting depending on the severity of his condition. However, it is vital for him to take his medication and visit his psychotherapist on time. Whenever possible, neighbors can also help to show some care and concern to make sure he takes his medications.

Living with Family or in a Hospital

It is advisable for a Schizophrenic patient to live with his family or in a hospital whenever possible. This is so that family members or medical professionals can keep track of the patient and make sure that he is taking his medications, attending group therapy sessions and meetings his psychotherapist on time. They can also keep track of the patient's behavior and see if it has improve over time.

A Schizophrenia patient who gets enough love, care and support from families are less likely to suffer from paranoid attack; it definitely makes it easier for him to live and cope with Schizophrenia.

Schizophrenia: Truth and Reality

Have you ever seen someone who talks about things that are out of this world? Have you encountered a person who talks like this? People with this behavior are sometimes diagnosed to have schizophrenia. Schizophrenia is considered as a challenging disorder, because when you are experiencing schizophrenia it is difficult to distinguish if things are real or unreal. It is also a brain disorder that affects the way a person acts, thinks and sees the world.

People with schizophrenia can see or hear things that don't exist, believing that someone will try to hurt them and feel like there is someone who is watching them. People who aren't affected with schizophrenia think that people with this illness are dangerous, however, most are not violent and dangerous at all. Most cases of schizophrenia appear in late teens or early adulthood. There are some rare cases of schizophrenia which appears in children but the symptoms are slightly different. It was also shown that the earlier schizophrenia develops, the more severe it is and it tends to be more severe in men than in women.

The causes of schizophrenia are not entirely recognized. Although, it shows that schizophrenia comes from the complex interaction between genetic and environmental aspects. It has a strong hereditary component but not all the families predisposed to schizophrenia develop the disorder. In environmental aspects, researchers believe that high levels of stress can trigger schizophrenia by increasing the body's production of the hormone, cortisol. Some studies also suggest that abnormalities in the temporal lobes and hippocampus are connected to schizophrenia's positive symptoms but even if there is an evidence of brain abnormalities, it is not true that schizophrenia is always the result of a problem in any particular region in the brain.

Sometimes schizophrenia appears suddenly and without warning but for most cases, it comes on slowly with warnings signs. The most common early signs of schizophrenia include depression, forgetfulness, inappropriate laughter or crying, deterioration of personal hygiene, suspicion, delusions, hallucinations, apathy, emotional unresponsiveness and social withdrawal. These warning signs can also results from a number of problems and not just schizophrenia. Aside from the warning signs, schizophrenia also has symptoms which vary from one person to another.

The symptoms are classified as positive symptoms, disorganized symptoms and negative symptoms. Negative symptoms refer to the absences of normal behaviors found in healthy individuals. Negative symptoms include blunted affect, catatonia and difficulties in speaking. Compared to the negative symptoms, the positive symptoms involve delusions and hallucinations, while the disorganized symptoms involve inappropriate emotional responses, lack of inhibition and a decline in overall daily functioning.

The symptoms of schizophrenia vary from one person to another and the treatment must be decided individually. Treatments include antipsychotic medications, electroconvulsive ("shock") therapy, psychotherapy, family support and rehabilitation. Antipsychotic medication has a greatly improved the outlook for people with schizophrenia. It reduces the symptoms of psychosis and usually allows a person to function more effectively. Neuroleptic is a typical antipsychotic drug that blocks the receptor in the brain of dopamine, which plays an important role in schizophrenia. However, an antipsychotic medication has side effects which include dry mouth, allergic reaction, weight gain, sexual dysfunction, menstrual irregularities and lethargy. Electroconvulsive therapy (ECT) also known as shock therapy is used to cause a low-voltage electric current and it is often suggested that it is safer than drug therapy but has falled out of favor recently. A psychotherapy session focuses on the current or past experiences, problems, thoughts and feelings. By sharing some experiences, people with schizophrenia will understand about the disorder and themselves. Rehabilitation may also be used in treating the disorder. It may aid a person regaining confidence to take care of themselves and have a productive life. Studies shows that people with schizophrenia will worsen in families who are hostile and emotional. However, it also shows that individuals improve when families are in self-help groups.

People with schizophrenia do not have split personalities rather they are split off from reality. Although it is a never-ending disorder, there is an aid available and the truth is, schizophrenia can be successfully handled. The first thing to do is to identify the signs and symptoms and seek help immediately. If the treatment is suited to the person they are more likely to stick with it. With the right treatment, therapy, medication and support from family and friends, the person with schizophrenia can have a happy and fulfilling life.

Schizophrenia - Do You Think You Have It?

There are several reasons and excuses for why Schizophrenia goes undiagnosed or mistreated. Sometimes it is the result of denial by the person affected with the illness, or by the people around them. Other times it is the result of lack of education about the illness and an inability to understand what the symptoms are. It is also possible that a Learning disability can be the direct effect of a bigger underlying mental illness issue that a medical professional has over looked.

These are just some of the reasons why Schizophrenia can go undiagnosed for years until something that is hard to explain occurs, such as a pyschoatic episode.

In the early stages of the illness, it is easy to say there is nothing wrong and choose to ignore the signs of the illness. It is very unsettling at the thought of having Schizophrenia and being diagnosed or labeled with it. But if left untreated or undiagnosed, Schizophrenia doesn't get better and will intensify with age. Fortunately, there have been medical advancements to help treat and manage Schizophrenia.It is an illness that you can count on it getting worse and depending on the severity, death could be the end result. Living with Schizophrenia that is untreated is a terrible way to live your life!

Denial of the Illness & why it is not Diagnosed.

I have a daughter that has Schizophrenia and in the early parts of her life, I knew as a mother that something was not right.There were many signs and things I noticed that were different, I would question them in my mind, touch on them with our family doctor, and then dismiss them saying, With time she would out grow these things.

I would fight with my husband all the time about her and his response would always be that she was just trying to get attention.When it did become evident that there was definitely something wrong, he still would not acknowledge that he had a daughter with any problems let alone an illness as debilitating as Schizophrenia. Even now my ex-husband still denies the fact he has a daughter with mental illness.

Denial is the number one reason why Schizophrenia is not diagnosed and why people do not seek help. Either denial by the person suffering or by the family around the person suffering, who denies it and says there is nothing wrong.

We all look for other possible non-severe reasons for a behavior. We tell ourselves lies, we think that it is our fault that things are this way, but they will get better over time. We say that time heals all wounds, but in this case, it will only get worse if not treated.

The second reason it is not diagnosed, is for the lack of information that is available about mental illness. For several decades, mental illness was never mentioned. For a long time it was not even taught in medical schools, let alone, mentioned in public information. We all thought of Schizophrenia as something that a psychopath had, because we would only hear about it when it was connected to a violent crime. In my mind, when I thought of mental illness, I thought of a person who was put away in an asylum and forgotten about, because you couldn't deal with them.

The fact is, in severe cases of mental illness, the person suffering can gravitate to the darker side of the mind. But as time passes and if they are not diagnosed, it is possible for these dark thoughts to become a reality for them and they may do something violent.

But if the illness is diagnosed early enough, then it is possible to treat and manage.

The symptoms of Schizophrenia may and can include:

Hallucinations (hearing voices, seeing people, seeing things that are not there) People with Schizophrenia can have varying degrees of this illness. Sometimes they will hear just voices and never seen anyone attached to the voice. Other times it is more severe and they will actually see people, creatures and things that are not there in reality, but to them they are very real.

Doctors call these hallucinations, but to a person with Schizophrenia, the voices and people that they hear and see are as real to them as you and I. People who are seeing or hearing these imaginary voices have a high tendency of talking out loud, becoming very vocal, and carrying on conversations with things that are not there.They will even turn music on really loud in their room so no one can hear them talking to these imaginary forces. They will lock themselves into their own room, to have these conversations where no one can hear them, and they can be left alone.

When you hear the mentally ill talking to someone or something that is not there, you get the sense that the conversation is happening with a real person, but there is no one in the room with them. Most of the time, if you ask them if they know the people they are talking to, they will typically say that they do not know they are. But, depending on what is going in their life, they may start to believe that they are seeing people who have passed away, or an actor that they saw on TV in a movie. Sometimes the people they choose to talk to in their mind, are strangers on the street that they walked by days or weeks earlier.

The problem with these hallucinations is that these interactions will often turn to a Dark Theme. They will start to talk or think about death, loss, evil, anger and fear. To some with Schizophrenia, the voices would verbally attack them about the person they are, and what they have done. They will say things like you are dumb, worthless, should never have been born and these dark comments and thoughts can continue to escalate to thoughts of harming themselves. The voices typically never stop and they are very distracting, judgmental, critical, and over bearing.

Delusions (false beliefs)

It is very hard to say to someone with Schizophrenia that the voices and people they see are not real. They can draw pictures of what they are seeing and can give you an exact recount of what is being said to them. But the reality is all these things that are being told to them, they will start to believe as absolute truth. One such example of this belief of the voices involves my daughter. The voices in her head told her that the food in front of her at meal times was poisonous and to eat it because they wanted her dead. If she did eat it, they would tell her that they are succeeding in killing her, and she would instantly throw it up.

As a result of this constant mental pestering, my daughter started to lose weight and became anorexic, and would not eat or keep food down. Because she believed what the voices told her about the food being poisonous, so she stopped eating.When the mentally ill start to believe the voices and people they see and hear, that is when the person you know, no longer acts and thinks the same way as they once did.

Even if you tell them over and over again that these voices are not real, they will not believe you. In their mind it is a perpetual dream or nightmare that never ends. But when you confront them about these voices that they consider to be absolute reality, they will start to become more secretive and will withdraw into their own world. Thus, shutting you out of their life as much as they can and it is almost impossible to reach them at that point.

Lack of Emotions or Inappropriate Display of Emotions

As the illness progresses, people with Schizophrenia become more and more withdrawn into this world of imaginary visions.

They hear and talk freely with the voices and they stop relating to reality. This disconnection from reality can and will result in loss of emotions, and inability to interact in the world. Once they have accepted this loss of reality, sometimes they start to believe that they have special powers that is given to them. Some of them believe they are receiving prophecies of what is to come, or they believe they are talking directly to god, angels, or the devil.Sometimes they believe that they have an important mission to do and no one else understands, so they need to keep it a secret.

Because they feel no one understands them, the typical day to day interactions with normal people will result by acting out with anger and frustration.

As I explained earlier, the illness does not get better if left untreated or undiagnosed. It will not improve as time goes on and they slip into their own self-made imaginary world.

They lose the desire to go to school, work, take care of themselves or do anything in life. Interactions with people can feel strained and stressful for them and they will choose to avoid people all together. They just want to be left alone to do what they feel they need to do. If they believe they have received a mission from the voices, then they just want to focus on that mission and forget about everything else.

Lack of motivation can be the direct result of a person with mental illness that is focusing entirely on the voices in their head. They will spend hours and days trying to decipher the supposed information they are being told.In several cases, what they are being told makes absolutely no sense to them, but they feel they need to do something to make the voices go away.

Trouble Functioning at School or in Social Situations

The constant nagging and pressure from these imaginary voices and people that pester the mentally ill is over whelming for them. As a result, they can become disorganized, easily distracted, an inability to focus or maintain consistent thinking.

They will act out inappropriately, say things in conversations that don't make sense, and laugh at things that are not funny. A complete social awkwardness. This makes functioning in school or social situations almost impossible for them.

For young adults and children, this type of social awkwardness can result in teasing and tormenting from people around them, making the illness even worse.

When this happens, they only want to disconnect from the world even more which will make it harder for them to function or fit in at school, work, or in social interactions.

Self-inflicting pain with the intent of a distraction from the voices and people they see.

Sometimes the constant voices in their head can be so overwhelming, that they just want it to stop and go away. In an attempt to get rid of voices, they will purposely injure themselves or cut their body to inflict pain. They will focus on the pain to push away the voices that they hear or the thoughts they have no control over. They will take extremely hot showers and try to focus on the hot sensation to draw their mind away from the voices.

They will drink or do drugs in attempt to shut out the voices to have some peace in their life. This is just a short list of the several ways a mentally ill person will deal with the imaginary world in their head. If any of these symptoms sound familiar to you or someone you know. Please take the necessary steps to get help.

Talk to someone you think will listen. Maybe your parents, friends, family member, or a Doctor. Explain to the best of your abilities what is happening to you and the specific things that are going on in your mind.People with mental illness can act very secretively and will keep a lot of things to themselves. They are very good at saying just enough to get by and not draw any attention to themselves. But with no treatment, after awhile it will become very obvious that something is not right.

They are afraid of what people may think about them, even worse they think that no one will believe them. In many cases, the voices in their head tell them that something bad will happen if they say anything. So they live in fear and will be scared of the possible repercussions of saying something. But the truth is, if the illness is not treated or diagnosed, the symptoms will only intensify. It will become harder and harder for the person suffering from the illness to function in the world. Eventually, the many secrets that they have been hiding from loved ones and friends will come out. But depending on the amount of time that has passed with no treatment it can result in several personal losses. Such as friends, family, work, school, and other loved ones in their life who do not want to be around them.

For Schizophrenia, the earlier it is diagnosed in life, the better chance a person has of living a normal and happy life. There is hope of living a normal life with Schizophrenia. But it is only possible through treatment and management of the symptoms with medicine and diagnosing it as early as possible. In my opinion, having a great caretaker is essential

OCD Schizophrenia - The Fact behind Differences and Similarities

Schizophrenia and Obsessive compulsive Disorder (OCD) are not alike. Yes, you've read it right. They are two different things but often co-occur with one another. Statistics show that approximately 15 out of 100 people who suffer from OCD also have schizophrenia. Schizophrenia is a grave mental sickness characterized by a gradual breakdown in a man's process of thinking and emotional awareness. This is believed to be influenced by risk factors such as heredity, depression, environment, drug addiction and a remarkable increase of dopamine levels in the brain. Signs and symptoms are typically manifested during childhood and young adulthood which include hallucinations, paranoid delusions, disorganized speech and catatonia. These in turn result in a person's both social and occupational dysfunction. Schizophrenia is being classified by health professionals into paranoid type, disorganized type, catatonic type, undifferentiated type, residual type, according to the individual's existing and presenting signs and symptoms. People who suffer from schizophrenia often have big troubles in establishing and maintaining both personal and public relationships. If the situation happens to get worse, hospitalization is often necessary.

OCD and Schizophrenia: Compared

While these two disorders equally affect both males and females they are often mistaken and interchanged, OCD as schizophrenia or schizophrenia as OCD. This is because obsessive compulsive disorder and schizophrenia have a lot of things in common and their manifesting signs and symptoms often overlap, same as with the concerned pharmacotherapy and the brain area being affected by both disorder. It is important to note, however, that many clinical studies show that those who suffer from OCD are less likely to develop schizophrenia, although those with schizophrenia are more likely to develop OCD.

In some cases, symptoms of OCD and schizophrenia may overlap adding to the difficulty of exploring and finding out the clear relationship between these two disorders. However, one significant manifestation of schizophrenia is the presence of delusions. Delusions are truly false irrational thoughts or beliefs contained by the sufferer even with the presence of strong evidences that suggests those are incorrect. While obsessions in OCD are usually associated with ideas of contamination, sexual impulses, symmetry or asymmetry, and hoarding things, delusions on the other hand are typically related to illogical thoughts of being a super hero with special powers and ideology associated with persecution wherein the individual with schizophrenia believes that whatever is happening around has always have something to do with him or her.

As it is difficult to diagnose the illness ourselves, it is much advisable to consult experts. Seeking help from a respected psychologist or psychiatrist would be better. They are the ones most eligible in finding natural, traditional, and modern techniues in the course treatment of OCD Schizophrenia.

Understanding the Various Effects of Schizophrenia on a Person's Life

Schizophrenia is a brain disease that affects the person's actions, thought processes and perception of reality. It is a difficult disease to foresee since schizophrenia happens not at a young age but in the late teen years to early twenty's for men and the late twenty's to early 30's for women.

What causes schizophrenia is not fully known but apparently there are linkages between genetic and environmental factors whose complex interaction may result in schizophrenia. Though genetics may play a role in this disease, it only determines one's predisposition to it, and not its development. More than half of people diagnosed with schizophrenia have family members who do not have that disorder. Like everything else, complications during pregnancy may have linkages to schizophrenia. Stress inducing conditions like low oxygen levels during the birthing process, a prenatal exposure to a viral infection and exposure to virus during infancy. It is believed that high levels of stress trigger the production of the hormone cortisol which as studies suggests, plays a role in schizophrenia. Another alleged cause of developing schizophrenia is brain chemical imbalances. Glutamate and Dopamine imbalances, as recent studies suggest, may contribute to schizophrenia. Abnormalities in brain structure may also cause this disease. CAT Scans taken from those afflicted by the ailment show enlarged brain ventricles which show a lack of volume and mass of brain tissue. Other possible contributors have to do with the measuring of brain activity from the frontal lobe which is responsible for the decision making, planning and reasoning processes.

These are some of the likely causes of schizophrenia and there are no definite conclusions but rather hypotheses of what may contribute to such an ailment.

The effects of schizophrenia are the ones most felt not just by the patient but by those around especially family members and friends. The biggest effect of schizophrenia is in the person's ability to interact with others. Since this ailment strikes at a later age, one can see a reversal of behavior. From a gregarious and communicative personality, one affected with this ailment can become withdrawn, and uncommunicative. Paranoia can set it which makes the person suspicious of everyone. Worse yet, one affected with schizophrenia may develop his or her language or become incomprehensible, offering uttering words that rhyme but not make any sense or even talking about things illogically. Such an effect of schizophrenia may lead to frustrations among both parties and immediate consultations with doctors are needed to help treat the ailment which is treatable with the appropriate medicine.

Advice For Getting Treatment For Schizophrenia

People are not born with schizophrenic symptoms. They can appear as early as age 16 or as late as 40 with the typical age around 19. If you feel that you are losing your mind or if your family and friends are showing concern that you have these problems that were listed in the introduction, be open to getting help.

Most forms of schizophrenia respond well to medications. Find a ⬚ualified psychiatrist to prescribe medications by calling your insurance or Google. If you do not have insurance many doctors will be willing to work a payment plan.

People with schizophrenia respond well to cognitive behavioral therapy. This is a therapy that includes examining your thoughts, choosing more appropriate and helpful thoughts and beliefs, and changing your behaviors to ones that will keep you safe and functioning well. Look online and find one in your area who treats schizophrenia. You can also call your insurance.

Your family and/or people you live with can be helpful. They can remind you to take your medications, they can guide you if you have a delusion or hallucination by gently helping you question it. You may wish to have one or more supportive people participate in a therapy session with you so the therapist can train them how to help you.

With schizophrenia you may always need to be on medication and you may need therapy or case management throughout your life. Sometimes you might be tempted to discontinue therapy or medication if you are faring well. Many people with schizophrenia lead happy and productive lives when they stay on their medication and get the help that they need.

Schizophrenia is an illness just like depression, anxiety, bipolar, the flu, etc. and it does not have to define who you are. You can look at what you are good at and what you are accomplishing in your life and see yourself as that and you happen to have an illness called schizophrenia.

When someone becomes aware that they have schizophrenia, they often think that they will never work, have a family, and do the things that others do. After receiving therapy for schizophrenia, often people can move from hospitalization to employment, marriage, and parenthood. It does not have to stop you from living a full and rewarding life.

People with schizophrenia have a behavior similar to people with depression and anxiety. They isolate themselves from the world, and from the people who could help them. Your family and friends can help you once they understand what you are going through.

Earlier in this book it mentions the ages of the onset of schizophrenia. If you are 19 years old or under 40 it is not necessary to worry about getting it. Often, people will get anxious that they have schizophrenia because they fall within the onset ages. There is no way to predict who will get it, so why worry?

Although you need medication and therapy, give yourself credit for being able to live a normal and successful life. It comes back to the idea that you are not schizophrenia, you are a person who has schizophrenia and you are also many other things.

There are many treatment options available for people with schizophrenia. You need to find a good psychiatrist and therapist and get support from the people in your life. Schizophrenia is a treatable condition that does not have to stop you from living your life to the fullest.

Alternative Medications for Schizophrenia

Schizophrenia is mental disorder that is thought to be an inherited condition that involves several different brain disorders. Medication is the most common treatment for this condition, but there are several different alternative and complementary treatments available for those seeking holistic treatment options. Alternative treatments include changes in diet, dietary supplements such as vitamins and herbs, and lifestyle changes.

Seeking Treatment

Schizophrenia is a very serious condition that can lead to harmful behaviors in those suffering from the condition. Because this disorder is serious, seeking treatment from an experienced physician is the first step in the process of recovery. Treatment with prescription medications allows those with schizophrenia to reduce symptoms while alternative treatments promote overall well-being and mental health. It is generally advised that patients with schizophrenia continue medications until a physician is consulted because there are often serious side effects when medications are suddenly stopped.

Types of Alternative Treatment Available

Alternative treatments for schizophrenia are focused on using dietary supplements, including herbs and vitamins, and making healthy lifestyle changes to encourage mental health. Drugs, such as marijuana, are harmful to patients and may make symptoms of schizophrenia more severe. Other steps toward health are also important. Reducing and eliminating alcohol and tobacco consumption are both steps toward healing holistically. Other treatments can safely be used with lifestyle changes. Therapy with a licensed therapist, using vitamins and dietary supplements, and attending group therapies are all options available.

Therapy and Schizophrenia

Therapy is widely accepted as being beneficial for anyone suffering from a mental disorder. Schizophrenia is now considered as a condition caused by chemical imbalances in the brain, but therapy can benefit patients with this disorder by allowing them space to work through problems and issues that arise in their personal life because of the disease. A psychologist can also provide resources that patients can use to encourage a healthy lifestyle. For instance, if rehabilitation services, such as group home living, is needed a therapist can provide recommendations.

Rehabilitation services are an important part of recovery after beginning a consistent medication schedule. Rehabilitation can include vocational and living training to assist patients in gaining the skills needed to live independently. Stress management skills are also important for those learning to live independently. Therapy and rehabilitation services are among the most important alternative therapies available for schizophrenic patients today.

Vitamins and Herbs

Modern therapies for schizophrenia can include the use of vitamin supplements or herbs to reduce the symptoms of the disorder and to improve overall health. It is important that patients check with a licensed physician before beginning the use of dietary supplements to ensure the herbal ingredients in supplements won't interact with any prescription medications currently being used. Some herbs have side effects and interaction precautions that make them unsuitable for use among schizophrenic patients. Vitamins are typically safe if taken according to the instructions on the label, but checking with a primary physician first is recommended.

One of the most common vitamins used in the treatment of schizophrenia is niacin along with Omega 3 fatty acids. This treatment is relatively safe. Some herbal treatments, however, can be dangerous when combined with traditional prescription medications. An alternative treatment for schizophrenia but the herb, when combined with medications, can result in lowered blood pressure.

Caution is important when using herbal treatments along with prescription medications. The most successful alternative treatments for schizophrenia are those that can safely and effectively be used in combination with traditional prescription medications. Advances in medical science have made prescription medications more effective and convenient for use than ever before. Medication, therapy, a healthy lifestyle, and rehabilitation services are the ideal combination of treatments available today.

How Does Schizophrenia Manifest?

When a child is diagnosed with schizophrenia parents are shocked because they can not understand how come a child that is intelligent, and looks good could be that ill.

Schizophrenia comes with symptoms just like any other disease but they differ from person to person. Some people might have just one episode of schizophrenia in their entire life, but in others schizophrenia might manifest more fre□uent and for a long period of time.

The first who notice there is something wrong with a person are the family members. They see that the person is not like it used to be any more and go for a check up at the doctor's.

Because schizophrenia gives perceptual difficulties the ill person might refuse contact with strangers and will isolate himself from others.

They will become less interested in their usual activities including work and personal hygiene and this will alert their family members that something is wrong.

Schizophrenia gives changes in personality at first only minor changes but after some time quite obvious changes. The inability of showing emotions like crying or laughing will install after a while and if they manage to laugh they make it in a strange way that makes it inappropriate. They become indifferent to others and to social activities and they end up isolating themselves.

A disorder in thoughts will install in most of the cases and the ill persons will not be able to concentrate as they used to and will forget a lot of things. They generally develop a problem with talking, they use odd language structures. They always seem confused and jump from a topic to another. Some might become hyperactive and will develop intense preoccupations with religion believing that they have a special mission, will write non stop meaningless phrases, and might use drugs and alcohol. Some develop extreme reactions to criticism and will even try to run away from home.

Due to the perceptual changes in their brain, the ill person might see, feel and smell things that are not there, that are not real. All these manifestations are hallucinations. In the worse cases they might attempt to suicide or to auto-mutilate because they seem to hear voices telling them to do that. All their senses are turned upside down and sometimes even a telephone ring might be confused for a fire alarm and provoke agitation among them.

The schizophrenic people realize that they have problems with their senses but they try to hide all the symptoms away, they will keep it a secret. They will deny all these facts and will avoid any situation that puts them face in face with the fact that they are different.

These ill persons are even more afraid that they will be abandoned by the loved ones and that is why family must always stand beside them and support them. All they need is love, patience and a lot of understanding.

Cigarette Smoking in People with Schizophrenia

For many years, it has been identified that patients with psychiatric illnesses like schizophrenia, smoke to excess. However, recent researches show that there has been a recurrence of interest in the high prevalence of nicotine addiction in people dealing with schizophrenic symptoms. It has turn out to be increasingly obvious that heavy cigarette smoking is closely associated with this psychological disorder and that this may have implications for the underlying neurobiology of the illness.

In people suffering from schizophrenia, the rate of smoking is believed to be between two and four times higher. Most schizophrenics who smoke take more cigarettes daily and smoke strong brands than the usual smokers.

Numerous studies and theories have been put forward as to why most people with this mental disorder smoke. Experts believed that nicotine acts as a form of self-medication for people suffering from schizophrenia, causing numerous beneficial effects despite the negative impact of smoking on long term health.

Smokers with schizophrenia report that the practice helps to reduce their symptoms. This has been confirmed by various studies proving that smoking is directly related to a reduction in the negative symptoms of the psychological disorder which include the lack of motivation, anxiety, and social withdrawal. Experts in schizophrenia believe that this effect is caused by nicotine's ability to increase dopamine levels in areas of the brain involved in awareness and interacting with the person's surroundings.

Clozapine which is considered as a kind of atypical antipsychotic drug that produce a reduction in negative symptoms, act in a similar way. On the other hand, there is no evidence that nicotine has an effect on positive symptoms of schizophrenia which involves abnormality in the affected person's content of thought. In addition, if nicotine is withdrawn from smokers with the mental disorder there is no increase in these symptoms.

Reduction of schizophrenia medication side effects is one of the reasons behind the excessive smoking of schizophrenics. Stiffness and rigidity of movement are examples of unpleasant side effects of antipsychotic drugs. Also, nicotine has also been found to work against the adverse side effects of antipsychotics medication on some kinds of mental function. A study of schizophrenics taking a typical antipsychotic drug called haloperidol that were given nicotine skin patches found them less affected by the unpleasant side effects.

The areas of the human brain involved in working memory, attention span, and motivation have a huge number of receptors for the nicotine molecule. Researches and studies show that nicotine develops these functions both in smokers with schizophrenia and non smoking people with the psychological disorder. However, people with schizophrenic symptoms usually display greater improvements than the general population. Also, there may be genetic differences that identify the extent to which an individual will be affected by the higher nicotine intake.

Given these negative effects of nicotine on a person's health, including the increased risk of heart disease and cancer, experts believe that there is an urgent need for treatments that provide the benefits of nicotine without the threats to long term health.

Schizophrenia Treatment - 5 Challenges to Cope with When Treating Schizophrenia

If your loved one suffers from schizophrenia, he, you and all of your family and friends are facing many challenges to cope with while treating schizophrenia. Here are 5 of the most significant challenges you are going to face during your treatment of schizophrenia:

1. Maintain a Daily Routine

If your loved one suffers from schizophrenia, it is going to be a difficult task to get him back to a daily routine. One that would make him occupied and not thinks about his illness all the time.

2. Being Active

When suffering from schizophrenia, your loved one is situated in a place that is being affected by the negative symptoms of schizophrenia and therefore suffers from a lack of energy and motivation to do stuff. How to ignite him and make him face the reality in an active manner is your real challenge as his loved one.

3. Being Independent

One of the most significant phases of having schizophrenia is lacking the ability to live by you. Therefore how to get him live his life in an independent way with his own protective environment, out of his parents' house is the real challenge.

4. Having his Own Income

This is another way to give your loved one the ability to live in an independent way as he should be. When that sufferer has his own job and income and not being dependent on the government support. When having your own money with out giving others a report about what to spend and what not to, is the real meaning of being independent.

5. Having Friends

When people suffer from schizophrenia, they are also suffering from relationships problems such as lack of friend or lack of his own mate. Therefore it is crucial to cause him to get new friends and even to find his own soul mate in order to be able to defeat his schizophrenia disorder.

Dealing With Schizophrenia - 5 Reasons for Having Children When Suffering From Schizophrenia

Whom we call healthy people, people who don't suffer from schizophrenia are usually taking the position of a moral police man and saying that it would be better if schizophrenia's sufferers won't have kids of their own. So as a contra to what they are saying, here are 5 reasons why schizophrenia sufferers should have kids of their own:

1. Better Education

It is well proven that people with schizophrenia give their children a better education in average, than people with out it. They get better manners, they are more sensible for their environments and they become better citizens to their country.

2. More Sensitive

Children to parents with schizophrenia, become more sensitive to their environment and to their surrounding people. They tend to be more mature compare to other normal kids. The reason is that they sometimes have difficult times with their suffering parents, and therefore they understand that life can be difficult sometimes.

3. Ready for Life

Children to parents with schizophrenia, become more ready to life than other normal children. As they went through one or two crisis in life, they become more resistant to life difficulties than other children. They are more mature than other in a way that helps them better deal with life challenges than others.

4. Less Violent

It has been proven that children to schizophrenia suffering parents become to be less violent grownups than other children. They are being raised in a calmer environment with less violence, what makes them in the long run better people with no violent tendencies.

5. Healthier

As a contradiction to the stigmatized point of view of other people, children of schizophrenia suffering parents, less tend to develop illnesses. But even if their chances to develop mental illnesses are higher, because of the other reasons that were mentioned before, we can predict that they would deal with their illness even better than their parents and therefore recover in a better and a healthier matter than other sufferers.

Don't let other people tell you what to do in the matter of having children or not. We prefer that people with schizophrenia would fulfill their basic instinct and human right of having children than becoming resembling to the darkest regimes that were and are controlling in some regions of the world through the history of man kind.

Conclusion

Schizophrenia is a disorder associated with high levels of social burden and cost, as well as an incalculable amount of individual pain and suffering. However, there is evidence that the outcome of care can be as successful as it is in many other diseases treated by medical or surgical procedures (National Advisory Mental Health Council).

Implementation of an effective care system for schizophrenia, however, is more than a technical endeavour. It has to be sustained by a vision and must be put within a unifying overall frame of reference. The vision can be that of a recovery-oriented mental health system, i.e. a service oriented to promote recovery from mental disorders by fostering self-esteem, adjustment to disability, empowerment and self-determination. Psychosocial rehabilitation can provide this vision with a frame of reference, linking mental health services to a complex and ambitious social perspective that encompasses different sectors and levels, from hospitals to homes and work settings, with a central aim of ensuring full citizenship for people irrespective of their disabilities (WHO).

In Conclusion, schizophrenia is a very complex mental disorder than can affect people with a variety of different symptoms. It has yet to be pinpointed exactly what causes this disease and what factors contribute to it, but it seems that genetics and environment play a crucial role inthe development of schizophrenia. There are different types of treatment options available for people that are dealing with this disease, including medication and/or counselling,